BASIC PSYCHOPHARMACOLOGY FOR COUNSELORS AND PSYCHOTHERAPISTS

BASIC PSYCHOPHARMACOLOGY FOR COUNSELORS AND PSYCHOTHERAPISTS

RICHARD S. SINACOLA, PH.D.

The Palm Springs Institute and Chapman University—Palm Desert

TIMOTHY PETERS-STRICKLAND, M.D.

Medical Psychiatric Associates of Delaware Valley

Boston ▪ New York ▪ San Francisco
Mexico City ▪ Montreal ▪ Toronto ▪ London ▪ Madrid ▪ Munich ▪ Paris
Hong Kong ▪ Singapore ▪ Tokyo ▪ Cape Town ▪ Sydney

Executive Editor: *Virginia Lanigan*
Series Editorial Assistant: *Scott Blaszek*
Marketing Manager: *Amy Cronin-Jordan*
Editorial Production Service: *Barbara Gracia*
Composition and Manufacturing Buyer: *Andrew Turso*
Electronic Composition: *Publishers' Design and Production Services, Inc.*
Cover Administrator: *Joel Gendron*

For related titles and support materials, visit our online catalog at www.ablongman.com

Between the time website information is gathered and then published, it is not unusual for some sites to have closed. Also, the transcription of URLs can result in typographical errors. The publisher would appreciate notification where these errors occurs so that they may be corrected in subsequent editions.

Library of Congress Cataloging-in-Publication Data

Sinacola, Richard S.
    Basic psychopharmacology for counselors and psychotherapists / Richard S. Sinacola, Timothy Peters-Strickland.
        p. cm.
    Includes bibliographical references and index.
    ISBN 0–205–44005–3
    1. Psychopharmacology. I. Peters-Stickland, Timothy. II. Title.

RM315.S56 2006
615'.78–dc22   2005047697

Printed in the United States of America

0 9 8 7 6 5 4 3 2 —09 08 07

In loving memory of
Jacqueline Palma Peroni-Sinacola, my mother,
and
Corrine Marie Sinacola, my sister

R. S. Sinacola

To my loving family
Howard, Alexia, and Alyssa

T. Peters-Stickland

CONTENTS

CHAPTER SEVEN
Treatment of Anxiety Disorders   51

CHAPTER EIGHT
Treatment of Psychotic Disorders   61

CHAPTER THIRTEEN
Treatment of Chemical Dependency and Co-Occurring Conditions   93

CHAPTER FOURTEEN
Treatment of Comorbidity and Other Disorders   101

CHAPTER FIFTEEN
Case Vignettes: Children   108

CHAPTER SIXTEEN
Case Vignettes: Adolescents   112

CHAPTER SEVENTEEN
Case Vignettes: Early Adulthood   117

Now more than ever, counselors and psychotherapists need timely information on the psychotropic medications that their clients are taking. Finding this information is not easy because most texts books on psychotropic medications are written by physicians for physicians. In the few cases where nonphysicians, usually biologically oriented PhDs, have attempted this endeavor, they have produced works that are more like a physiological psychology text, which are beyond the basic questions and interests of the student, counselor, or psychotherapist.

Basic Psychopharmacology for Counselors and Psychotherapists is designed to provide basic, yet comprehensive information for both the typical graduate student in a counseling, social work, marriage and family therapy, or psychology program, and the practicing clinician in the field. Most graduate students have not taken an undergraduate course in physiological psychology, and their knowledge of the brain and neuronal functions are minimal. This textbook presents these and other topics in easy-to-understand language. In fact, the entire text is written in a familiar style that invites the otherwise intimidated professional to learn more. Medical jargon is kept to a minimum and voluminous information on psychopathology is also omitted, because we assumed that clinicians and graduate students are familiar with the *The Diagnostic and Statistical Manual of Mental Disorders*, 4th ed.-TR (DSM-IV) and the criteria used in diagnostic determinations.

In addition to offering up-to-date information on the medications currently available for treating mental illness and other related conditions, this book will also assist clinicians in working more effectively with their patients on medication and with the professionals prescribing them. The book is organized to address the most commonly seen types of pathology first.

- Chapter 1 gives both students and their professors and practicing clinicians reasons why the study of psychopharmacology is so important for the mental health professional.
- Chapter 2 provides a basic explanation of the functions of the brain and neurological system, including the anatomy and function of neurons, the role of neurotransmitters and other neurochemicals involved in emotions and behavior, and the electrical and chemical communications between cells.
- Chapter 3 addresses issues related to psychopharmacology and pharmacokinetics including methods of administering drugs; absorption, distribution and elimination of drugs; therapeutic dose and therapeutic index; tolerance, withdrawal, and discontinuance of drugs; synergism and potentiation; placebo effects; and prescription and pharmaceutical terms.

- Chapter 4 provides the therapist with both tools and techniques for taking a thorough history of the patient including a patient history outline, a mental status outline, assessment and testing instruments, and an outline for an initial patient interview.
- Chapters 5 through 12 address trade and generic medications and herbals used to treat common mental health conditions: unipolar depression; bipolar illness; anxiety and psychotic disorders; ADHD and attention disorders; and cognitive, sleep, and personality disorders.
- Chapter 11 is an entire chapter on sleep disorders that was included because many clinicians who deal with patients presenting with these concerns are unfamiliar with the medications used to treat insomnia.
- Chapter 13 addresses chemical dependency and co-occurring conditions and the special medications used to treat this population. This topic is not addressed in most other texts.
- Chapter 14 provides typical medication regimes used to treat patients with co-morbid conditions including patients with chronic pain, eating disorders and obesity, impulse control problems, sexual compulsivity, and other intrusive behaviors.
- Chapters 15 through 19 present cases across the developmental continuum including children, adolescents, early adulthood, middle adulthood, and older adulthood patients. Many of the cases are based on actual patients. The cases are used to demonstrate both the diagnostic process and the rationale for choosing one medication over another.
- Complete, yet easy-to-read, tables of medications appear throughout the text and are combined into a master table in the Appendix.

This text serves as a basic introduction to psychopharmacology for the non-medical provider. While information on dosage and use was accurate at the time of writing, the clinician should not use this information as a guide for prescribing medications. All clinicians should consult their respective codes of ethics and their home state's scope of practice to insure that discussing medications and their effects with patients is within the scope of their license to practice.

This book was designed to be a brief, yet concise, overview of clinical psychopharmacology. It can be read easily in a weekend and will serve as a handy reference guide for mental health professionals from all disciplines. Combined, we have over thirty-five years of clinical experience as a psychologist, who both conducts a private practice and teaches psychopharmacology in a graduate setting, and a psychiatrist, who treats patients from all walks of life. We hope that the reader finds this book both informative and interesting.

We wish to acknowledge the editors and staff at Allyn and Bacon for their help and encouragement in completing this task.

We would also like to thank the following reviewers for their time and feedback in making this book a worthwhile contribution to the field:

Matthew R. Buckley, Delta State University
Darlene G. Colson, Norfolk State University
Katherine Dooley, Mississippi State University
Patricia Goodspeed, SUNY Brockport
Thomas J. Hernandez, SUNY Brockport
Joy P. Kannarkat, Norfolk State University
John M. Morgan, Humboldt State University
Jodi Ann Mullen, Oswego College
Curtis D. Proctor, Wichita State University

R. S. Sinacola, PhD
Palm Springs, CA

T. Peters-Strickland, MD
Pennsylvania, PA

ABOUT THE AUTHORS

Richard S. Sinacola, Ph.D., is a licensed psychologist and director of The Palm Springs Institute and Alternative Health Services in Palm Springs. He was the former Chair of Counseling and Addiction Studies at the University of Detroit Mercy. He is now Core Professor of Psychology at Chapman University—Palm Desert. In addition to teaching, Dr. Sinacola is a senior lecturer and trainer for PESI Healthcare Corporation. He has served on the editorial board of the Michigan Journal of Counseling and Development, and he is the past secretary of the Michigan Psychological Association. He lectures internationally on various mental health topics. He holds degrees in psychology, counseling, and clinical social work from The University of Detroit and Wayne State University.

Timothy Peters-Strickland, M.D., is a psychiatrist with Medical Psychiatric Associates of Delaware Valley in Philadelphia, Pennsylvania. Dr. Peters-Stickland has held an appointment as a clinical instructor with the University of Southern California. He is a diplomat of the American Board of Psychiatry and Neurology with an added qualification in Addiction Psychiatry.

BASIC PSYCHOPHARMACOLOGY FOR COUNSELORS AND PSYCHOTHERAPISTS

CHAPTER ONE

WHY STUDY PSYCHOPHARMACOLOGY
Reasons for the Nonmedical Therapist to Read This Book

Over the years various counseling and psychotherapy models have emerged, flourished, continued, or faded from use. Many of these theories or models offered the clinician options for maximizing the therapeutic progress of their client. Many of them emphasized humanistic, psychoanalytic, or behavioral techniques that downplayed the role of medication in the treatment of many conditions. In fact, except for those patients with serious psychopathology necessitating inpatient hospitalization, most patients were not on medications and therapists liked it that way!

Today, a vast majority of the patients seen in private practice settings and in community mental health agencies either have been, are, or will be on psychotropic medications. Most therapists, however, have not received additional education to keep pace with a changing treatment arena. In fact, most nonmedical therapists—namely, psychologists, social workers, professional counselors, and marriage and family therapists—have never taken a course in psychopharmacology and feel ill prepared to handle patients and clients on psychotropic medications.

Some therapists choose not to seek this information. They offer the argument that they work with cancer patients and do not need to know the etiology or how to treat it. This argument has some truth in it, however, it might not be a valid premise for choosing to be naive on the topic. For example, it has been well documented that all therapists need to be aware of the role physical illness plays in mental illness. If any ethical or professional therapist or counselor feels that a physical condition might be a cause for a patient's condition, the therapist should immediately refer the patient to a physician for an evaluation. Amazingly many do not! While it might be true, that once a physical condition is treated it often disappears. In the mental health field, treatment is often a combination of psychotherapy and medication. As a mental health *expert*, the clinician is expected to diagnose and treat various conditions and be aware of the best treatment for them. To choose to exclude a large part of the treatment protocol is, if nothing less than limiting, a disservice to the patient. Therapists who claim that medication is not part of their approach with patients because it interferes with their therapeutic work are often lulled into a false sense of inclusiveness. In their world the only way to treat a patient is with nonmedical therapy, and if the patient is not responding, then he or she is resisting.

For years psychiatrists have been accused by nonmedical therapists of being pill pushers. These therapists often site the refusal of psychiatrists to spend any "real therapeutic time" with patients as evidence that the psychiatrists either lack therapeutic skills or view everything as a medical issue. The truth here is that many nonmedical practitioners feel uncomfortable talking to psychiatrists and other prescribers about medications. Many nonmedical practitioners choose to reduce every psychological concern to purely behavioral manifestations and refuse to even consider the role of biology or neurology. This choice is not new even among nonmedical therapists. Some social workers and even nurses have minimized the need for psychological testing with clients only because they do not perform these services. Many were afraid to refer clients to psychologists for psychological testing, because they feared that the psychologist might steal their client. Turf wars between psychologists and psychiatrists have also lead to issues of who is the "real" doctor in charge of the case. In many states both the physician and the psychologist share hospital privileges. Additionally, some states and jurisdictions allow properly trained psychologists, clinical nurse specialists, and physician assistants to prescribe medications.

Many nonmedical therapists agree that knowledge of psychotropic medications is necessary and attempt to gain this knowledge, yet they still feel inadequate when it comes to their level of knowledge. They still refuse to discuss medications with clients and defer always to the "doctor." These therapists may claim that they do not wish to practice medicine without a license. Many therapists, such as licensed psychologists, are aware that their scope of practice allows them to discuss medication options with patients, but they are not necessarily the person who may ultimately prescribe them. Still, these therapists claim ignorance and defer any decisions. They may be unclear as to what role they should take with patients regarding their medications.

One analogy may fit here. Consider the patient a consumer who has a car that is not functioning properly. She may not be sure what's wrong with the car, so she takes it to a local repair facility (mental health clinic). The mechanic (therapist) is well trained in how to listen to the engine and determine the problem. He will then suggest a plan of repair (treatment). In many cases he knows where the problem is and how to fix it, but he may not know why the problem occurred or why the part failed. The engineer (the physician) may be able to offer an explanation here. She knows what the part was designed to do, and why it physically failed. She may also be able to fix the part if it is taken to the factory (hospital). If the car needs to be redesigned, the engineer, not the mechanic, would attempt to do it. A therapist who has no knowledge of psychotropic medications is like a mechanic who listens to the car and says, "Yep, you have a problem all right, and I think it's in the transmission. Maybe you want to see an engineer."

In reality, most good mechanics and dealerships employ engineers and structural technicians who work together to repair your car. In the same way, therapists and physicians need to work together in the best interests of the patient.

How does a nonmedical therapist or counselor determine just what they need to know? Consider the following quiz:

1. **What is an SSRI?**

    If you said an antidepressant, you get one point. But do you know that SSRI stands for selective serotonin reuptake inhibitors? Do you know the primary neurotransmitter involved in their action? Do you know the major side effects? Can you name the six major drugs in this class by brand name? Would you recognize the chemical names if you saw them in a medical record? If a client told you a doctor placed him on meds and he was having side effects A, B, and C, would you know that the side effects came from the SSRI?

2. **What is a neuroleptic?**

    If you said a medication for treating schizophrenia, you get another point. But do you know the primary neurotransmitter that is involved in their action? Do you know the side effects? Do you know which medications are major tranquilizers and which are minor? Do you know which medications are better for the negative symptoms of psychoticism?

3. **What is a benzodiazepine?**

    If you said they are used to treat anxiety you once again get a point. But do you know where they interact in the brain? Do you know what neurotransmitter or amino acid is involved? Are they habit forming? Can someone overdose on them?

If you were able to answer all of the above questions correctly, you do not need to read this book and could probably teach others about psychopharmacology. If you knew a few answers, consider reading further and you will not be disappointed. If you knew none of the answers, definitely read on.

This book will assist the nonmedical therapist increase his or her knowledge base of medications and their proper use. Without complicating the picture with excessive biological terms and neurochemistry, it will give the counselor only the necessary information to work safely with a patient currently taking or considering medications. It will also offer helpful suggestions to therapists working directly with psychiatrists and other prescribers.

CHAPTER TWO

BASIC NEUROBIOLOGY

This chapter will provide basic information on the purpose and function of the brain's neurological system with regard to mental-health functioning.

Topics to be addressed include the following:

- Neurons
- Neural communication
- Electrical and chemical properties of neural transmission
- Neurotransmitters of emotion and behavior

As a counselor or psychotherapist, you will need to understand how the brain works to control thinking, behavior, and overall health. Further knowledge in this area should assist you in comprehending your client's symptoms and disease process. The field of psychopharmacology is evolving rapidly and will continue to change with advances in medical research. New interventions to treat psychiatric illnesses should enhance the quality of life for your mental-health clients.

This chapter provides some basic information on which to build an understanding of various medications, their mechanisms of action, and how they might be used in day-to-day practice. This chapter describes the anatomy of nerve cells or neurons, how they fit together, and the ways they communicate.

NEURONS

Since the brain is the most complex organ in the body, the discussion here will be limited to neurons in the central nervous system and the effect of drugs on it. Within the central nervous system, neurons transmit messages or communicate with each other, and as you will learn later, drugs can affect this transmission. In order to understand how messages are transmitted, you must first understand how a neuron is structured.

A neuron has four basic parts: the soma, dendrites, axon, and terminal buttons (see Figure 2.1).

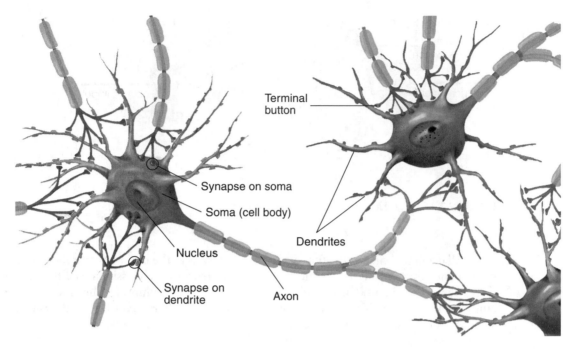

FIGURE 2.1   The Structure of a Neuron

- The *soma*, or cell body, contains the vital parts of the cell, including the nucleus, mitochondria, and other substances in the cytoplasm (the space inside the neuron). A membrane defines the boundary of the cell.
- *Dendrites* are large and small branches of the neuron, similar to branches of a tree, that receive messages from other neurons through multiple molecular receptors.
- The *axon* is a long slender tube that carries messages from the soma to its terminal buttons.
- *Terminal buttons* are found at the ends of branches of the axon. They contain small sacs, or vesicles, that hold chemical messengers, or *neurotransmitters*. Terminal buttons deliver neurotransmitters to other neurons across a physical gap called a *synapse*. The synapse can be between a terminal button and a dendrite or between a terminal button and the soma.

NEURAL COMMUNICATION

Within the central nervous system, neuron communication is facilitated either electrically or chemically. This communication is facilitated electrically within the neuron and chemically between neurons.

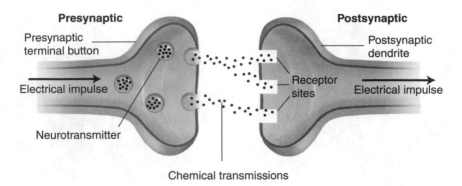

FIGURE 2.2   **Electrical and Chemical Communication Between Cells**

All drugs and substances that can activate neurons in the brain or central nervous system and, thus, affect communication between neurons are classified as either endogenous or exogenous. *Endogenous* substances, such as endorphins, insulin, and adrenalin (also known as ephinephrine), come from within the body. *Exogenous* substances, such as caffeine, vitamins, herbs, and medications, are produced outside the body and introduced into the body in some manner.

Receptor sites on the postsynaptic membranes of dendrites are often the targets of medications that can activate adjacent cells. That action begins when a receptor is stimulated by a neurotransmitter. Once stimulated, an electrical impulse travels along the axon toward the terminal button. Because an electrical signal or impulse is unable to cross the synapse, the transmission of the signal across the synapse depends on chemical messengers, or neurotransmitters. After the electrical impulse reaches the terminal button, a neurotransmitter is released. It travels from the presynaptic membrane of the terminal button across the synapse to the postsynaptic membrane of another neuron's dendrites where it might interact. The postsynaptic membrane of the dendrite contains numerous receptors that receive the chemical signal and, in turn, activate the postsynaptic cell, allowing it to transmit again (see Figure 2.2).

ELECTRICAL AND CHEMICAL PROPERTIES OF NEURAL TRANSMISSION

The electrical properties of a neuron relate to the difference between intracellular (inside the cell) ion concentrations and extracellular (outside the cell) ion concentrations; ions are electrically charged molecules. The most common ions found in the extracellular spaces are sodium (Na^+) and chloride (Cl^-) ions. The most frequent intracellular ions are potassium (K^+) and negative protein ions. The *resting potential* of a neuron is the unexcited or relaxed state where the average electrical difference between the inside and outside of the cell is about 70 millivolts (mV). The resting potential is usually referred to as −70 mV (the outside is more negative than the inside).

Other electrical properties that affect a cell include depolarization and hyperpolarization. When a cell is stimulated or *depolarized*, it fires an electrical message that is called an *action potential*. An action potential is produced when a neuron's resting potential becomes less negative or depolarized. After an action potential occurrs, the cell briefly becomes more polarized or *hyperpolarized* before it returns to a relaxed state. A depolarized membrane is more likely to transmit an electrical impulse; a hyperpolarized membrane is less likely to transmit an electrical impulse.

When neural transmission occurs, the signal may be excitatory or inhibitory in nature. Excitatory messages increase the likelihood that an electrical impulse will be sent; inhibitory messages decrease that likelihood. All neurons may receive both excitatory and inhibitory messages at the same time. Whether a message is or is not transmitted depends on the relative number of excitatory and inhibitory signals a neuron receives. For example, if the excitatory messengers outnumber the inhibitory messengers, an action potential (message) will be initiated along the axon.

All action potentials are the same size when they are generated, but not all behavioral responses are equal in magnitude. More significant, or stronger, environmental stimuli produce a higher number of action potentials (a higher rate of firing of action potentials). The higher the rate of firings of action potentials, the stronger we would expect the behavioral response. For example, a loud sound may generate ten action potentials in a time period, whereas a soft sound may generate only two action potentials during the same period. Thus, the behavior response to the loud sound is usually greater than the response to the soft sound.

When the action potential reaches the nerve terminal, neurotransmitters are released by a process called *exocytosis*, the secretion of a substance by a cell (see Figure 2.3). At the end of the axon, the action potential causes calcium ions (Ca^{++}) in the terminal button to release vesicles of neurotransmitter into the synapse. The neurotransmitter then diffuses across the synapse to interact with receptors on the postsynaptic membrane of the dendrites or soma. When receptors are activated, ion channels, or little gateways, open on the postsynaptic membrane causing either depolarization or hyperpolarization. An excitatory signal leads to the process occurring again; an inhibitory effect decreases further signals. Remember that depolarization excites and hyperpolarization inhibits. The action potential is officially over when some of the neurotransmitter is taken back into the terminal button in a process called *reuptake* (see Figure 2.4).

A neurotransmitter and its individual receptor site is like a key fitting into a lock (see Figures 2.5). Receptors, located on the extracellular membrane, are specific types of protein structures made of amino acids. The structures make each receptor unique. By a process known as *signal transduction*, the first messenger or neurotransmitter binds to a receptor that transmits the message by changing the electrical characteristics of the cell, by starting a biochemical action within the cell, or both. (The second messenger will be explained later.) In general a neurotransmitter may open an ion channel in either of two major ways. One direct way is through ligand-gated, ion-channel receptors (neurotransmitters and drugs are generally referred to as ligands). An ion channel opens when a ligand binds to the receptor site (see Figure 2.6). In turn, the influx of particular ions leads to either depolarization or hyperpolarization. For example, the acetylcholine receptor works in this manner. When two acetylcholine molecules

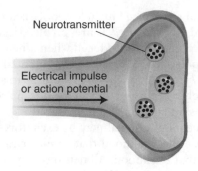

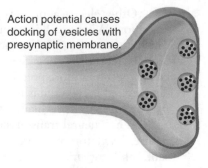

Stage 1: Axon potential travels along axon to terminal button.

Stage 2: Action potential causes vesicles to fuse with presynaptic membrane.

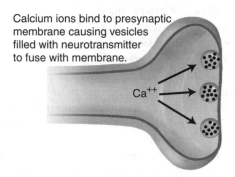

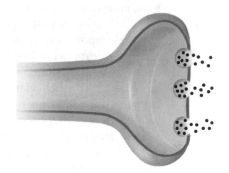

Stage 3: Action potential causes calcium ions to release vesicles of neurotransmitter into synapse.

Stage 4: Neurotransmitter released into synapse.

FIGURE 2.3   The Four Stages of Exocytosis

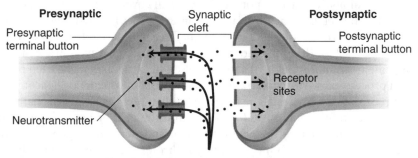

Reuptake pumps or transporters remove the neurotransmitter from the synaptic cleft via the terminal buttons. This terminates the action potential.

FIGURE 2.4   The Process of Reuptake

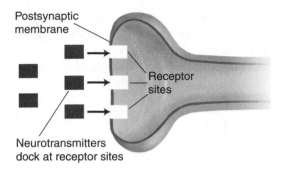

FIGURE 2.5   Receptor Sites

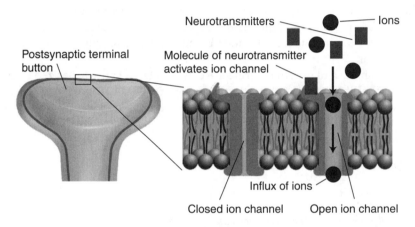

FIGURE 2.6   Ion-Channel Activation

occupy the two acetylcholine sites on a single receptor, a sodium pump is opened, resulting in an influx of sodium (Na$^+$) ions that causes depolarization.

The second way a neurotransmitter opens an ion channel is by inducing chemical changes within the cell. The majority of receptors that produce these effects are called G protein-linked receptors because they bind guanine nucleotides. For example, dopamine, glutamate, gamma-aminobutyric acid (GABA), and serotonin all facilitate neurotransmission by utilizing G protein-linked receptors.

After the first messenger or neurotransmitter interacts with the extracellular receptor, the chemical effects of the G proteins activate a second messenger within the cell. The most well-known second messenger is cyclic adenosine monophosphate or cyclic AMP. Thus, the neurotransmitter or first messenger binding to the receptor causes a cascade of chemical reactions in the postsynaptic neuron involving a second messenger. Cyclic AMP usually activates other molecules or enzymes that in turn break down other chemicals. The resulting substances are known as protein kinases. The protein kinases facilitate a change in the physical shape of other proteins that control the opening of an ion channel. The alteration in the physical shape of the protein permits the channel to open, allowing an influx of ions into the postsynaptic neuron. This ion influx causes either depolarization or hyperpolarization. The final results of this process vary but may include making other neurotransmitters, sending further electrical charges, and so on. An increasing complex cascade of effects occurs that alters cellular function.

NEUROTRANSMITTERS OF EMOTION AND BEHAVIOR

Three main neurotransmitters involved in emotion and behavior are the catecholamines (dopamine and norepinephrine) and one indolamine (serotonin). The category designation catecholamine or monoamine is based upon chemical structure. Other neurotransmitters that might be considered include three important amino acids: GABA, glycine, and glutamate. In addition, certain chains of amino acid known as neuropeptides, including substance P and endorphins, may play a role in emotion and behavior.

Dopamine and norepinephrine are closely related and synthesized from the same precursor substance known as tyrosine (see Figure 2.7). Tyrosine is an amino acid that comes from diet. Synthesized tyrosine can be purchased in a health food store, how-

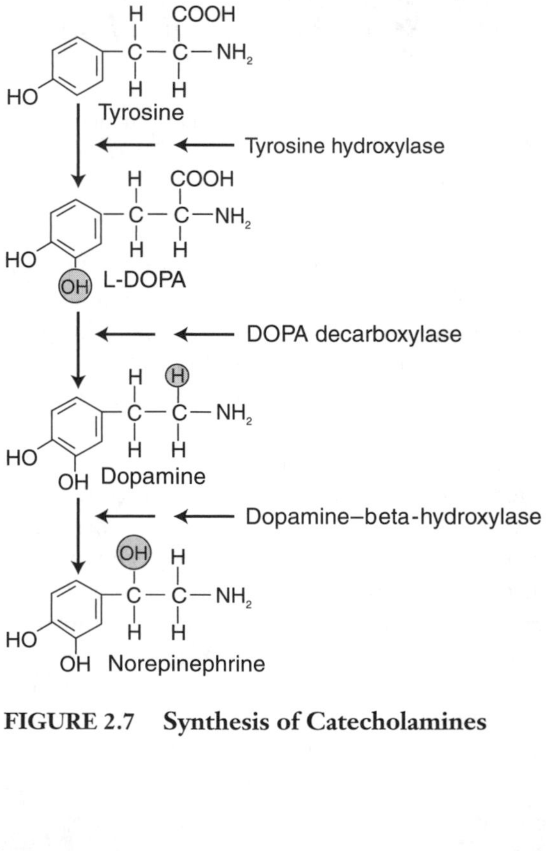

FIGURE 2.7   Synthesis of Catecholamines

ever, it has not been shown to be as effective as tyrosine obtained from a food source. Dietary sources of tyrosine include meat, poultry, seafood, beans, tofu, and lentils. Tyrosine enters dopaminergic neurons by diffusion, where the cytoplasmic enzyme tyrosine hydroxylase converts it to L-DOPA. L-DOPA is then converted by DOPA decarboxylase into dopamine. Some of the dopamine may be further converted by dopamine β-hydroxylase into norepinephrine.

The noradrenergic (or norepinephrine) pathways in the brain seem to be involved in regulation of sleep-wake cycles, sustained attention, alertness, and biological responses to new stimuli. Noradrenalin is also thought to mediate anxiety, fear, and stress responses. Thus, noradrenergic abnormalities or drops in norepinephrine levels are thought to play a large role in mood and anxiety disorders.

Serotonin or 5-hydroxytryptamine (5-HTP) is synthesized from tryptophan in our diet (see Figure 2.8). Once again, synthesized tryptophan supplements have not been shown to be an effective way of obtaining serotonin. Dietary sources of tryptophan include bananas, sunflower seeds, and milk. Tryptophan is converted into 5-hydroxytryptophan by an enzyme called tryptophan hydroxylase. Then 5-hydroxytryptophan decarboxylase acts on 5-hydroxytryptophan to produce serotonin or 5-hydroxytryptamine.

Scientists believe that serotonin plays a large role in brain functioning including mood, anxiety, arousal, irritability, tranquility, cognition, appetite, sleep-wake cycles and obsessions. Serotonergic abnormalities or drops in serotonin levels are associated with anxiety disorders, mood disorders, and even psychotic disorders. Explanations of neural activity might seem quite concrete and straightforward but the systems are much more complex. Neurons have an extraordinary number of diverse interconnections. Because behavior is complicated, no one neurotransmitter should be considered in isolation, that is, an individual's depression might be caused by insufficient levels of serotonin, norepinephrine, dopamine, or in some cases, all three. Most brain functions

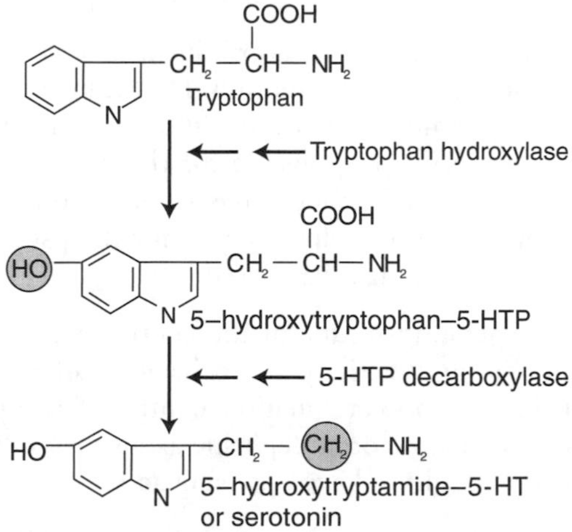

FIGURE 2.8   Synthesis of Indolamines.

result from multiple influences of several different neurotransmitters trying to find their own delicate balance.

Drugs may alter behavior by interfering with or interrupting any of the processes that occur during neural communication. A drug that increases the availability or action of a neurotransmitter is called an *agonist*. For example, fluoxetine (Prozac) increases the action of serotonin on the postsynaptic membrane. Conversely, a drug that decreases the availability or action of a neurotransmitter is called an *antagonist*. For example, risperidone (Risperdal) blocks dopamine at the postsynaptic membrane. Keep these concepts in mind. They will be revisited in later chapters with respect to specific diseases and medications.

In summary, a few neurotransmitters are particularly important for those in the mental health field. The following gives you a general foundation for each one.

■ *Acetylcholine.*   In the central nervous system, acetylcholine is widely distributed and thought to play a role in memory, learning, behavioral arousal, attention, mood, and rapid-eye movement activity that occurs during sleep. In the peripheral nervous system, acetylcholine is found at synapses where the nerve terminals meet skeletal muscles, causing excitation leading to muscle contraction.

■ *Epinephrine or Adrenalin.*   This neurotransmitter is probably more active in the peripheral nervous system rather than the central nervous system. Epinephrine is secreted by small endocrine glands above the kidneys known as the adrenal glands. In the peripheral nervous system, epinephrine regulates our "fight-or-flight" response. Its role is described in Chapter 7, The Treatment of Anxiety Disorders.

■ *Norepinephrine.*   Primarily, norepinephrine is an excitatory neurotransmitter in the central nervous system. Norepinephrine cell bodies in the brain stem have axons projecting into the limbic system (brain structures involved in emotions) and the frontal lobes. Wakefulness and alertness are the two major functions of norepinephrine. The role of norepinephrine is discussed later in Chapters 7 and 9.

■ *Dopamine.*   Another major neurotransmitter, dopamine is involved with behavioral regulation, movement, learning, mood and attention. Dopamine may have both excitatory and inhibitory effects in the brain. It is belived that overactivity of dopamine or oversensitivity of dopamine receptors is responsible for the major symptoms in schizophrenia. Amphetamines, cocaine, and other drugs of abuse directly activate dopamine receptors. The resulting excitation helps account for the psychotic symptoms that are commonly seen when these drugs are abused.

■ *Serotonin.*   Another major neurotransmitter in the central nervous system is serotonin, which involves the inhibition of activity and behavior. Other areas where serotonin plays a significant role include mood regulation, control of eating, sleep and arousal, and pain regulation. Serotonin and norepinephrine axons project into almost the same areas of the brain and are thought to have opposing actions.

■ *Other Neurotransmitters.*   By virtue of its inhibitory nature, GABA makes the brain more stable by decreasing the neural transmission that prevents over excitation.

Benzodiazepines and barbiturates are two good examples that act to increase GABA. (See Chapter 7 for more about GABA.) Glycine is another inhibitory amino acid neurotransmitter that is present mostly in the spinal cord. When glycine receptors are activated, the cell becomes hyperpolarized and less likely to transmit a signal. Strychnine, a toxin that causes convulsions, acts by blocking these glycine receptors, leading to over-excitation and possibly death. Glutamate, another amino acid neurotransmitter, is definitely excitatory. More neurotransmission occurs because glutamate lowers the threshold for neural excitation. Glutamate is often found in Asian food in the form of monosodium glutamate (MSG), which excites the taste buds on the tongue (for further reading see Carlson (2004).

CHAPTER THREE

PSYCHOPHARMACOLOGY AND PHARMACOKINETICS

This chapter will address issues related to psychopharmacology and pharmacokinetics, how drugs work and bring about chemical and behavioral changes in the body, and how drugs are dispensed and prescribed. It will provide some basic information that is helpful in understanding the patient.

Topics to be addressed include the following:

- Routes of drug administration
- Drug absorption, distribution, and metabolism
- Other pharmacokinetic principles
- Therapeutic index dose
- Tolerance and withdrawal
- Discontinuation syndrome
- Potentiation and synergism
- Placebo response
- Prescription and pharmacy terms.

When we talk about pharmacology and more specifically psychopharmacology, we need to start with some basic concepts. In Chapter 2, Basic Neurobiology, we described *pharmacodynamics*, which may be defined as the study of how drugs affect receptor sites, send signals, and cause some neurochemical changes. On the other hand, *pharmacokinetics* refers to the administration, absorption, distribution, metabolism, and elimination of a drug inside the body.

ROUTES OF DRUG ADMINISTRATION

Medications may be introduced into the body by various methods including orally (by mouth), subcutaneously (deep tissue injection), intramuscularly or IM (muscle injection), intradermally (dermal injection), intranasally (nasal spray), inhalational (respiratory infusion), sublingual (dissolution under the tongue), transdermally (skin absorption), and intravenously or IV (venous injection). The most common way that a drug is administered is by mouth or orally. In recent times, there are a few medications delivered orally in the form of a "soltab" or orally dissolving tablet. Many psychiatric drugs are introduced into the body in this way. Examples of soltabs include: olanzepine (Zyprexa Zydis), mirtazepine (Remeron Soltabs), risperidone (Risperdal M-tabs), and clonazepam (Klonopin Wafers).

In more acute settings such as a hospital or clinic, intramuscular injections are commonly used to control behavior. Long-acting intramuscular injections such as haloperidol (Haldol Decanoate), fluphenazine (Prolixin Decanoate), or risperidone (Risperdal Consta) are used for more chronically mentally ill patients.

DRUG ABSORPTION, DISTRIBUTION, AND METABOLISM

Drug Absorption

When a drug is introduced orally, the rate of absorption is determined by the form of the drug. For example, liquids are absorbed faster than capsules or tablets. Over the last few years, many slow- or extended-release forms of medications have become available. They allow for fewer doses per day and fewer side effects because of the slower rate of absorption. Oral administration gives the slowest rate of absorption when compared to intramuscular, intravenous, and the other forms available. Absorption usually occurs in the stomach and duodenum (the first segment of the small intestines). Some medications need to be given with food for better absorption; some need to be given without food, which might interfere with absorption. Some gastrointestinal diseases and their treatments may also interfere with drug absorption, for example, antacids interfere with certain antibiotics.

Drug Distribution

After administration and absorption into the venous system, drugs are delivered throughout the body by the circulatory system. The liver is the first organ that orally absorbed drugs encounter. It will breakdown some of the drug into nonactive metabolites. This process in the liver is known as the *first-pass metabolism*. After leaving the liver, the drug is delivered to its target organ. The central nervous system is the target for psychotropic drugs. Other factors that affect drug absorption include: protein binding, drug half-life, and lipid solubility.

Protein Binding.   Some drugs bind tightly to plasma proteins such as albumin in the bloodstream. This *protein-binding* phenomena determines how much drug is available to act on the brain. Drug protein binding also hinders a drug's metabolism and excretion, which causes it to remain in the circulatory system longer.

Drug Half-Life.   The *half-life* of a drug is the average time required to eliminate one-half of the drug's concentration. For example, alprazolam (Xanax) has a half-life of 11 hours. Thus, the concentration of alprazolam will be reduced by about 50 percent after 11 hours, by 75 percent after 22 hours, and so on. In general, it takes approximately five half-lives for any drug to be eliminated completely from the body.

Lipid Solubility.   The *lipid* or fat *solubility* of a drug determines how easily it crosses a cell membrane, which is important for absorption and effectiveness at its target site. Drugs that are more lipid soluble (lipophilic) will cross membranes easily and are more likely to cross over the blood-brain barrier. Some drugs will not cross this barrier and do not exert their effects on the central nervous system.

Drug Metabolism

In ways that can get very complex, drugs are metabolized or broken down primarily in the liver by the *P450* family of *enzymes*. These enzymes are important because of the potential for drug interactions when multiple drugs compete for the same pathways. The liver breaks down the drug into other forms or metabolites that are later excreted in the urine. Geriatric patients have decreased liver enzyme activity that requires drug dosages to be reduced to avoid toxicity. Other medical conditions such as viral hepatitis or liver cirrhosis might also decrease a drug's metabolism. A few of the psychiatric medications, such as lithium, are not metabolized by the liver and are excreted unchanged by the kidneys in urine. A patient with kidney dysfunction may not excrete the drug normally, and the concentration may become elevated or toxic.

OTHER PHARMACOKINETIC PRINCIPLES

Therapeutic Index and Dose

The concept of *therapeutic index* is pharmacokinetic principle that needs to be addressed. When a certain drug concentration gives a desired response, it is referred to as a *therapeutic dose*. When a drug concentration causes mild or severe side effects, it is referred to as a *toxic dose*. The difference between a drug's therapeutic level and its toxic level is referred to as the *therapeutic index*. Desirable drugs have a high therapeutic index because the risk of toxicity at therapeutic doses is minimal. On the other hand, drugs that have a low therapeutic index carry more risk because the therapeutic concentration is relatively close to its toxic level. For example, lithium is difficult to use because the toxic level is slightly higher than the typical therapeutic level (see Chapter 6 for further details).

When determining a drug's therapeutic dose, it might be helpful to consider a dose-response curve (see Figure 3.1). When a drug is introduced into the body, a slow titration upward of the dose usually corresponds to an increasing response. This effect is true up to a certain point when the response of the drug levels off despite significant increases in the drug dose. As you might expect, increasing the drug's dose at this point only increases the risk of side effects and toxicity. Although most medications are introduced slowly into the body, some drugs may be initiated at high doses in order to

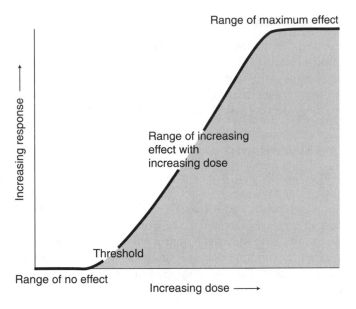

FIGURE 3.1   Dose-Response Curve

obtain a certain desired response. We call this a *loading dose* of the medication. After *loading* the patient, further dosage adjustments are seldom needed because we have introduced the therapeutic dose into the body all at once.

Tolerance and Withdrawal

Two important concepts that need to be defined are tolerance and withdrawal. The *tolerance* of a drug is defined as needing greater amounts of a drug over time to produce the desired effect. *Withdrawal* of a drug is defined as characteristic symptoms that emerge when a drug is abruptly discontinued after heavy and prolonged use. Depending on the substance, withdrawal symptoms can be medically dangerous and require inpatient hospitalization. Tolerance and withdrawal are relatively easy to understand when considering alcohol. Tolerance to alcohol develops over time, causing a person to increase the amount he or she consumes to obtain the desired effect. Withdrawal from alcohol develops when "an alcoholic" suddenly stops drinking, thus throwing his or her body into a state of shock. This withdrawal causes an expected array of symptoms such as tremors, agitation, insomnia, hallucinations, and even seizures. Tolerance and withdrawal are terms commonly used when working in the field of chemical dependency or addictions. In the DSM-IV, addiction is more specially defined as substance abuse and dependence. Addiction is discussed in Chapter 13, Treatment of Chemical Dependency and Co-Occurring Disorders.

Discontinuation Syndrome

A relatively new concept in the field of psychopharmacology is the *discontinuation syndrome*. This syndrome is distinct from withdrawal because it is not medically dangerous although some people claim that they are going through withdrawal. For example, patients who take paroxetine (Paxil) often report that when they miss a dose or stop taking the medication, they feel malaise and other flulike symptoms.

Potentiation and Synergism

A therapist must understand the concepts of potentiation and synergism. *Potentiation* means that one drug may enhance the effect of a second drug. For example, drug X added to drug Y may potentially cause drug Y to be more sedating. One drug that potentiates another drug may only increase the sedation effect by 2-fold or so. *Synergism* refers to the fact that one drug may significantly enhance the effect of a second drug by more than expected. For example, drug X added to drug Y may increase the sedation effect of drug Y by 6-fold. Because of synergism, a patient should not mix alcohol with benzodiazepines.

Placebo Response

A discussion about psychopharmacology and pharmacokinetics would not be complete without mentioning the *placebo response*. During any patient interaction, a complex series of events and communications occur in addition to any prescribed drug effects. Some patients will respond regardless of the specific therapeutic intervention just because of a helper's "therapeutic interaction" with them. Many patients have shown actual chemical changes in their brain when they receive a placebo even when an actual drug is not present. The brain acts "as if" the drug were present even though the medication is not. The power of the placebo response should never be underestimated.

PRESCRIPTION AND PHARMACY TERMS

Therapists will encounter numerous Latin abbreviations when reviewing records, prescriptions, and discussing issues with their prescribing professional (see Table 3.1). Although these abbreviations seem quite foreign at first, they become familiar with use over time.

It is always good practice to record a patient's medication regime in his or her chart. This information might be necessary when consulting with other professionals involved in the patient's care. Chapter 4 describes history taking and assessment techniques in further detail.

TABLE 3.1   Latin Abbreviations

ABBREVIATION	MEANING	LATIN
a.c.	before food	ante cibum
b.i.d.	twice a day	bis in die
cap.	capsule	capula
c with bar on top	with	cum
h.	hour	hora
hs	at bedtime	hora somni
p.c.	after food	post cibum
p.o.	by mouth	per os
p.r.n.	as occasion requires	pro re nata
q4h	every 4 hours	quaque 4 hora
q6h	every 6 hours	quaque 6 hora
qd	every day	quaque 1 die
q.i.d.	four times a day	quater in die
Rx	prescription	recipere
stat.	immediately	statim
tab.	a tablet	tabella
t.i.d.	three times a day	ter in die

CHAPTER FOUR

HISTORY TAKING AND ASSESSMENT TECHNIQUES

This chapter reminds the clinician that good history taking is essential to a good diagnosis, and a good diagnosis is essential before any referral or recommendation for medication.

Topics to be addressed include the following:

- Obtaining patient history
- Mental status examination
- Patient questionnaires and assessment instruments
- Structuring the initial interview

OBTAINING PATIENT HISTORY

No mental health professional should underestimate the importance of good history taking. It is always important to inquire about a patient's physical health before starting any counseling relationship, especially when a patient presents with issues of depression, anxiety, psychoticism or other highly intrusive behavior. By getting all of the facts surrounding a presenting issue, a therapist is assured that all relevant contributing factors have been considered.

It is critical to take a thorough history from a patient and to use assessment instruments that address the issue the patient presents. Depending on the setting where the history is taken, a few simple questions on the presenting problem, nature of concern, history of the problem, relevant family history, physical findings, and history of treatment might be sufficient. If time allows, however, a more detailed assessment may be in order. The following outline provides a detailed history and assessment of the patient.

Patient's History Format

I. Identifying Information
Name, age, sex, race, grade, religion, marital status, occupation and diagnosis (if applicable)

II. Presenting Problem
   a. Chief complaint
   b. How he/she was referred to you
   c. Dates of treatment or assessment
   d. How the person defines the problem
   e. Duration, intensity of concern (history of presenting problem)
   f. Any history of counseling/therapy

III. Personal/Family History
   a. Grandparents, parents or other relatives
   b. Spouse, lover and his/her relationship with them
   c. Children, stepchildren, and the relationship
   d. Siblings and the relationship
   e. Friends and the relationship
   f. Religion or other spiritual beliefs
   g. Complete school history (grade, H.S. or college)
   h. Present career status and beliefs about work
   i. Physical health/chronic illnesses
   j. Sexual history or concerns
   k. Any cultural or environmental issues

IV. Summary of Psychometric Information
   a. Summarize the results of any test instruments used. Be sure to mention the type of test, norms, and all scores collected.
   b. If you are interpreting test results administered by another professional, be sure to state all observations as quotes and compare with your findings.
   c. Accurately summarize reports from other sources such as family and friends. Give reasons for obtaining this source of information.

V. Diagnostic Assessment
   a. Present a developed, logical summary of the status of the patient. This summary should include a mental status exam, the clinician's observations and conclusions of the patient's level of functioning. Be sure to comment on the patient's intellect and maturity level.
   b. Assess the patient's coping abilities and comment on ego strengths and defense mechanisms.
   c. Give an example of the patient's insight level and his/her strengths and weaknesses.
   d. Make a complete diagnostic statement including an appropriate DSM-IV-TR, multiaxial diagnosis.

VI. Proposed Treatment Goals and Methods
   a. Be sure that all goals and methods relate to the diagnostic assessment.
   b. Define the goals and the objectives leading to them.

    c. Differentiate between short- and long-term goals.

    d. Describe the length and frequency of sessions.

    e. Describe the theoretical approach used.

    f. Describe special issues during treatment, for example, transference, counter-transference, or ethical issues.

    g. List other resources or professionals utilized (psychiatrist, nurse, psychologist, social services, etc).

    h. List referrals made to other professionals or agencies.

    i. Evaluate the treatment approach.

    j. Describe complete prognosis.

VII. Other Information

    a. Describe special circumstances encountered.

    b. Mention releases needed for consults.

MENTAL STATUS EXAMINATION

It is wise to obtain a baseline measure of mental status from all patients. This information not only gives a snapshot of how the patient is doing, but it gives a general sense of the patient on several different realms including cognitive capacity, intelligence, memory impairment, abstract reasoning, and judgment. If done properly, a good mental status can help to predict a patient's behavior and provide valuable information for making a diagnosis. A full mental status should include information from the following sources:

Mental Status Information

Attitude and Behavior
- Describe appearance including hygiene, makeup, and dress.
- Describe mannerisms: lethargic, hyperactive, echopraxia, posture, etc.
- Describe attitude toward self and others.
- Describe affect: sad, flat, labile, etc.

Stream of Mental Activity
- Describe flow of speech: tangential, rapid, spontaneous, blocked, etc.
- Describe language deviations: clang associations or echolalia.

Emotional Reactions
- Describe displays: tearful, anxious, flat. Congruent with stated mood?

Mental Trend and Thought Content
- Describe major themes of conversation
- Describe evidence of auditory, visual, gustatory, tactile, olfactory, or visceral hallucinations
- Describe delusions, ideas of reference, paranoia, or grandiosity
- Describe somatizations, suicidal, or homicidal ideation
- Describe history of substance abuse and list of current medications.

Sensorium, Mental Grasp and Capacity
Ask questions to determine the following:

■ Oriented X 3 (person, place, and time)
■ Memory: Immediate (recall of three items after five minutes); recent (events of last evening); remote (name last nine presidents)*
■ Calculations: Serial 7s and 3s; digits forward and backward
■ General intelligence and similarities: Abstract reasoning and proverbs

General Fund of Knowledge
■ Ask questions of common knowledge and current events and of items that assess past academic achievements.

Judgment and Insight
■ Ask questions to assess the patient's common sense (ego strengths) and ability to live independently.

A typical narrative description for the findings of the mental status exam would be worded in the following fashion, depending on the particular questions asked of the patient and his or her level of cooperation:

> Mrs. Jane Doe is a 30-year-old, African-American female of average height and weight. Her hygiene and dress were appropriate for the evaluation. She was oriented X 3, and while her speech appeared normal, she began to stutter when she became nervous. She denied hallucinations or other psychotic manifestations. Memory appeared intact with good immediate, recent, and remote memory. She appeared to have no educational or learning deficits. The patient appeared to have an above-average level of intelligence. She denied suicidal/homicidal ideation and chemical dependency.

PATIENT QUESTIONNAIRES AND ASSESSMENT INSTRUMENTS

For therapists, including those who are not psychologists, several patient checklists and questionnaires are available that can be used for patients who present with depression and/or anxiety. These instruments are designed to be user friendly for both the clinician and the patient. While some psychometric knowledge is helpful, most of these self-report format instruments are designed to be administered by mental health professionals with at least a master's degree and some relevant clinical experience. Some assume that the clinician has special training in their use, and may require the practitioner to be a licensed psychologist. A test's publisher may require professional credentials before selling the instrument. The following list is by no means exhaustive, but it represents some popular tools used in the field today. To learn more about them,

---

*If patient is from another culture/country, they could list their last four leaders.

type in the name of the test as a keyword on the Internet for publisher and research information.

Assessments for Depression

- The Beck Depression Inventory II: Twenty-one items, easy to score
- The Hamilton Depression Inventory: Available in a 17- or 21-item format; better for assessing somatic, less cognitive-related depression
- The Geriatric Depression Inventory: Helpful to use with an older population

Assessments for Anxiety

- The Beck Anxiety Inventory: Brief, easy to score, and helpful in differentiating between generalized anxiety and panic disorder
- The State-Trait Anxiety Inventory: Helpful in determining if the anxiety is one of an emotional reaction "state" versus more of a personality "trait."

General Assessment of Personality Including Depression, Anxiety, and Other Manifestations

- The Minnesota Multiphasic Personality Inventory (MMPI-2): Consists of 567 true/false questions over 10 clinical scales including depression, somatization, anxiety, antisocial tendencies, paranoia, mania, and psychoticism. Also available in an adolescent version (MMPI-A).
- The Million Clinical Multiaxial Inventory-III: Shorter with 175 items; better for assessing the presence of a personality disorder
- The Personality Assessment Inventory: Consists of 344 items; shorter version called the PAS or Personality Assessment Screener contains only 22 items and takes less than six minutes to administer

STRUCTURING THE INITIAL INTERVIEW

When a patient presents for counseling services and the therapist is aware that the patient may be in need of medication to treat a serious, affective anxiety, or thought disorder, it is very important to gather as much information as possible. The following are information-gathering suggestions to keep in mind.

1. Take the name of the patient's primary care physician (PCP) and the date of his or her last history and physical. Be sure to include any information on known diseases such as hypertension, diabetes, cancer, stroke, thyroid conditions, and so on. If the patient does not have a PCP, then he or she should be referred to one for a work-up as soon as possible. Be sure to ask the physician to assess for thyroid function, glucose tolerance, and electrolyte imbalances. Typical tests would include complete blood count (CBC), thyroid function tests, a basic metabolic panel, and urine toxicology.

2. Take a complete history of any treatment for the presenting problem. This history should include the types of symptoms, that is, depression, panic, anxiety and so on. Be sure to include all professionals the patient has seen and any medications he or she has taken. Ask the patient, are the medications helpful, effective, or intolerable? What side effects, if any, did you experience and did they lead to noncompliance?

3. Prepare a complete mental status using other assessment instruments as appropriate to confirm initial impressions. It would be appropriate for the therapist to formulate some initial short-term goals for proceeding with this patient.

Good treatment starts with a good history and assessment. Taking a few extra moments with the patient to address the above mentioned issues will assure both the patient and the therapist that no stone was left unturned. Be sure to review the treatment plan with the patient to confirm that he or she is also in agreement. By knowing the patient's history, the therapist can save time later by not reexposing the patient to medication regimes that did not work or that interacted with other medications the patient was taking for a medical condition. Pleading ignorance or claiming not to be a physician is no protection from a malpractice claim. Always remember that you are treating the whole patient.

CHAPTER FIVE

TREATMENT OF UNIPOLAR DEPRESSION

In this chapter we will examine the medications and other treatment considerations for patients with depression. Depression is the most common presenting concern in all treatment settings. Assessing the nature and type of depression is key to proper medication suggestions.

Topics to be addressed include the following:

- Biological versus environmental depression
- Causes of biological depression
- Counseling and psychotherapy
- Medications for depression
- Herbal and holistic substances
- Light therapy for seasonal affective disorders (SAD)
- Importance of exercise
- Electroconvulsive therapy (ECT)
- A step approach to patient treatment

BIOLOGICAL VERSUS ENVIRONMENTAL DEPRESSION

Depression is probably the most frequently presented issue in any mental health setting. Researchers have estimated that at any one time, at least 3 percent of the population suffers from chronic depression. More than 17 percent have had at least one episode in their lifetime, and another 10 percent reported an episode in the last twelve months (Sutherland, Sutherland, & Hoehns, 2003). It is interesting and sad that with all of the recent advances in both psychotherapy and medications for depression, only 30 percent of those with depression seek treatment for the condition (Rakel, 1999). In addition, less than 20 percent of those who seek treatment take antidepressants (MacIntyre, Muller, Mancini, & Silver, 2003).

Therapists have many issues to consider when treating depression. First, they must determine the nature of the depression. Some forms of depression are biological or *endogenous* in nature; they are said to be caused from *within* the person. This form of depression is likely to have a biological link or perhaps a family link to others who also have depression. In fact, Rakel (1999) mentions that monozygotic twins have a 65 percent concordance rate, and dizygotic twins have a 14 percent rate. Some forms of depression are more reactive or *exogenous* and are typically caused from forces *outside* of the body. In these cases, stress or grief may be the cause. Therapists often find that both internal and external factors play a role in many patients' depression.

It is important for the therapist to determine the nature and source of a patient's depression. At times it may be rather clinical or endogenous in nature. Typically, major depression and the depressive phases of bipolar conditions meet these criteria, but therapists are also aware that dysthymia, cyclothymia, and grief reactions have some biological components. Further, the clinician must determine the role of other complicating factors such as substance use, psychotic features, physical diseases, and medications that may cause depression.

CAUSES OF BIOLOGICAL DEPRESSION

For many patients presenting with depression, the cause can be related to another physical disorder that they may have. The following is a list of diseases and disorders that can cause or exacerbate depression:

Addison's disease	Diabetes mellitus	Multiple sclerosis
Alzheimer's disease	Fibromyalgia	Myocardial infarction
Anemia	Hepatitis	Pancreatitis
Asthma	HIV—AIDS	Parkinson's disease
Brain tumor	Huntington's disease	Porphyria
Cancer	Hyperthyroidism	Postpartum hormonal changes
Cardiovascular conditions	Hypothyroidism	
Chronic fatigue syndrome	Influenza	Premenstrual dysphoric disorder
	Lupus	
Chronic infections	Malnutrition	Rheumatoid arthritis
Chronic pain syndrome	Menopause	Stroke
Colitis	Mental retardation	Syphilis
Congestive heart failure	Metabolic abnormalities	Tuberculosis
Cushing's disease	Mononucleosis	Uremia

In addition to the diseases and disorders mentioned above, many medications and other substances have been known to cause or worsen a patient's depression. The following is a list of these medications and substances:

- Alcohol
- Antianxiety medications: diazepam, chlordiazepoxide, alprazolam, lorazepam, clonazepam, phenobarbital
- Antihypertensive medications: reserpine, propranolol, methyldopa, guanethidine sulfate, clonidine, hydralazine, metoprolol, prazosin
- Anti-inflammatory medications: indomethicin, butazolidin, rofecoxib (withdrawn from U.S. market in 2004), celecoxib
- Antiparkinsonian medications: levodopa/carbidopa, amantadine
- Cold remedies: antihistamines, others containing alcohol
- Corticosteroids and other hormones: for example, estrogen, progesterone, cortisone acetate, most oral contraceptives
- Drugs of abuse: marijuana, codeine, morphine, PCP, crystal methamphetamine, psychedelics, opium derivatives, synthetic pain killers
- Sedative-hypnotic medications: zolpidem, zaleplon, triazolam, flurazepam, temazepam, meprobamate

If after careful history and assessment, the therapist determines that the patient's depression appears to have little or no physical cause, a treatment plan is proposed to address the concern. While it is a well-known fact that psychotherapy and counseling alone are very effective treatments for depression, psychotherapy and medication together are most efficacious (Segal, Kennedy, Cohen, & Group, 2000). In cases of dysthymia (chronic-mild depression), psychotherapy alone may be attempted. If little response is noticed, an antidepressant may be added. In cases of a grief reaction with sleep disturbances, medications to improve sleep may be used without an antidepressant. Only when the grief is prolonged, severe, and accompanied by suicidal ideation, should antidepressants be considered. Suicide assessment is very important to keep in mind, as up to 80 percent of depressed patients also have suicidal ideation (Sonawalla & Fava, 2001). The following is a list of treatment options for the patient with moderate to severe depression.

- Counseling and psychotherapy
- Medication, including pharmaceuticals and herbal remedies
- Light therapy for those with seasonally influenced depression
- Exercise
- Electroconvulsive therapy (ECT) and other treatments

COUNSELING AND PSYCHOTHERAPY

Psychotherapists often underestimate the effective nature of therapy. However, psychotherapy as a medical treatment has been found to be more effective than by-pass surgery, drug treatments for arthritis, and even aspirin for heart attack (Lipsey & Wilson, 1993). Further, research on the percentage of improved patients at selected sessions has demonstrated that patients typically show the greatest gains in the first 16–20 sessions (Howard, Kopta, Krause, & Orlinsky, 1986). While nearly every form or approach of counseling or psychotherapy is helpful, some therapists believe that solution-focused therapy or briefer forms of therapy offer quicker solutions. Still others believe that cognitive-behavioral approaches work better than other forms (Rakel, 1999).

MEDICATIONS FOR DEPRESSION

For the most part, antidepressants can be divided into four main categories: tricyclic antidepressants (TCA), selective serotonin reuptake inhibitors (SSRI), monoamine oxidase inhibitors (MAOI), and heterocyclics or "others."

The oldest classifications of antidepressants are the TCAs. Tricyclic antidepressants have been around for more than forty years. They prevent the reuptake of neurotransmitter substance back into the presynaptic cell. Although effective, TCAs are not "clean" medications, and therefore, they affect many nontarget organs and systems in the body. They have troublesome anticholinergic side effects that include sedation, weight gain, difficulty urinating, dizziness, dry mouth, sexual dysfunction, orthostatic hypotension, and blurred vision. Typically these medications are not safe for children or the elderly. Due to their toxic cardiovascular nature, TCAs pose a serious risk of overdose for patients with significant suicidal ideation.

As was mentioned in Chapter 2, a patient's depression may be caused by depletions in the neurotransmitters serotonin (5-HT), norepinephrine (NE), dopamine (D) or all three. Table 5.1 lists TCAs with their trade and generic names, typical daily doses, neurotransmitter action, and level of sedation.

TABLE 5.1   Tricyclic Antidepressants (TCAs)

TRADE NAME	GENERIC NAME	TYPICAL DOSE (MG/DAY)	NEURO-TRANSMITTER 5-HT	NEURO-TRANSMITTER NE	LEVEL OF SEDATION
Anafranil	clomipramine	100–250	***	*	Heavy
Ascendin	amoxapine	150–400	*	***	Moderate-heavy
Elavil	amitriptyline	150–300	***	*	Heavy
Ludiomil	maprotiline	150–225	***	0	Moderate
Norpramin	desipramine	150–300	0	***	Light
Pamelor, Aventyl	nortriptyline	75–125	**	***	Moderate-heavy
Sinequan, Adapin	doxepin	150–300	**	***	Heavy
Surmontil	trimipramine	100–300	**	**	Moderate
Tofranil	imipramine	150–300	***	**	Light-moderate
Vivactil	protriptyline	15–60	*	***	Light

*Minimal neurotransmission, **Moderate neurotransmission, ***Significant neurotransmission

In the early 1980s, a second-generation drug was introduced with the trade name Desyrel and the generic name trazodone. This medication affects primarily serotonin but acts more as a 5-HT2 receptor antagonist. Trazodone is less likely to cause sexual side effects but may cause priapism, a condition resulting in a prolonged, painful erection, in men. Overall it has fewer side effects than older TCAs and is less of a suicidal risk, but the typical side effects of sedation and dry month remain. Less expensive generic TCAs are available making this medication more affordable for many patients. Trazodone is often used as a general sedating medication without the risk of addiction to sedative hypnotics for those who have trouble sleeping.

In the late 1980s, a new generation of drugs was born. Selective serotonin reuptake inhibitors, or SSRIs, block the reuptake of serotonin back into the presynaptic cell. This blocking action allows more serotonin to exert its influence on the postsynaptic cell. Table 5.2 lists SSRIs, their trade and generic names, typical daily dose, and level of sedation.

The side effects for SSRIs are considerably less severe than for older TCAs. Typical side effects include headache, nausea, diarrhea, dry mouth, anorexia, weight gain, restlessness, insomnia, tremor, sweating, yawning, dizziness, inhibited sexual desire, and inhibited orgasm for some. As mentioned earlier, SSRIs are "cleaner" and interact with few other medications the patient may be taking. They are considered safer medications for children, seniors, and patients who may be at risk for a suicide overdose; however, recent FDA warnings suggest that 2 to 3 percent of children and adolescents will demonstrate an increase in suicide thinking and behavior (see the FDA website, www.fda.gov). Many clinicians believe that the benefits of SSRIs outweigh their risks, because without treatment, severely depressed children and teenagers are at serious risk of suicide. If serotonin levels inside the central nervous system become too elevated from SSRIs or other medications, some patients may experience *serotonin syndrome*. Symptoms may include agitation, confusion, insomnia, flushing, fever, shivering, muscle rigidity, hyperreflexia, incoordination, diarrhea, and hypotension. Many of theses symptoms can be life threatening, therefore, any patient started on medication for the first time should be closely monitored.

TABLE 5.2   Selective Serotonin Reuptake Inhibitors (SSRIs)

TRADE NAME	GENERIC NAME	TYPICAL DOSE (MG/DAY)	LEVEL OF SEDATION
Celexa	citalopram	10–60	Light
Lexapro	escitalopram	5–20	None
Luvox	fluvoxamine	50–300	Light
Paxil, Paxil CR	paroxetine	20–50/25–50	Moderate-heavy
Prozac, Sarafem	fluoxetine	20–80	None
Prozac Weekly	fluoxetine	90 (weekly)	None
Zoloft	sertraline	50–200	None

In the last few years, heterocyclic antidepressant medications have been introduced that fall into the "other" category. These medications offer many possibilities (see Table 5.3).

Heterocyclic antidepressants have side effects similar to SSRIs, but they have less possibility of sexual dysfunction. Venlafaxine (Effexor/Effexor XR), a serotonin-norepinephrine reuptake inhibitor (SNRI), is usually well tolerated and has been shown to be helpful in general depression, generalized anxiety, and postpartum depression (Cohen, 1997). It has been known to increase blood pressure at higher doses. Duloxetine (Cymbalta), released in 2004, is similar to venlafaxine as a result of its dual mechanism of action. Duloxetine has the advantage of allowing for stimulation of both serotonin and norepinephrine equally at all doses. Venlafaxine is more serotonergic at lower doses.

Mirtazepine (Remeron) is helpful in restoring normal sleep patterns. It has also been found to increase appetite, which is an undesirable side effect for overweight, depressed patients. However, because of this side effect, mirtazepine may work wonders in depressed HIV or cancer patients who are having trouble with weight loss. Like mirtazepine, nefazodone (Serzone) may help restore sleep patterns and cause sedation for many. Unfortunately, the medication has an FDA "black-box" warning due to its increased risk of liver failure and must be used only with caution.

Bupropion (Wellbutrin) is well tolerated but is rather uplifting and agitating for some. While bupropion has not been associated with sexual dysfunction, it is not appropriate for patients with seizure or eating disorders, as it lowers the seizure threshold and reduces appetite.

The last major classification of antidepressants is known as monoamine oxidase inhibitors or MAOIs. These drugs work a bit differently than the others. They inhibit MAO or the enzyme that breaks down neurotransmitters and renders them ineffective. MAOIs exert most of their influence in the presynaptic cell. While the side effects of MAOIs closely resemble those of TCAs, MAOIs are usually well tolerated. Patients taking MAOIs must adhere to strict dietary restrictions, as ingestion of any food containing tyramine may cause a hypertensive crisis. MAOIs have fallen out of use in this country but are still widely used in Europe. Many prescribers use them as a last-resort drug for patients who do not respond well to other medications. (see Table 5.4).

In order to be comprehensive, lithium must be mentioned as a possible treatment option for unipolar depression as well as for bipolar depression. This strategy is usually reserved for more difficult and treatment-resistant cases. Lithium will be explored further in Chapter 6.

HERBAL AND HOLISTIC SUBSTANCES

St. John's wort is a plant that is said to have medicinal properties. Research, primarily conducted in Europe, claims that St. John's wort helps to control mild to moderate levels of depression with virtually no side effects (Bloomfield, Nordfors, & McWilliams, 1996). Most practicing clinicians believe that few patients are helped by St. John's wort, and they are now learning that it may interfere or react to other medications patients may be taking. For example, St. John's wort potentiates blood

TABLE 5.3 Heterocyclic Antidepressants

TRADE NAME	GENERIC NAME	TYPICAL DOSE (MG/DAY)	NEURO-TRANSMITTER 5-HT	NEURO-TRANSMITTER NE	NEURO-TRANSMITTER DA	LEVEL OF SEDATION
Cymbalta	duloxetine	20–60	***	***	0	None
Effexor	venlafaxine	50–300	***	***	*?	None
Effexor XR	venlafaxine XR	75–300	***	***	*?	None
Remeron, Remeron Soltab	mirtazepine	15–45	***	***	0	Heavy
Serzone[1]	nefazodone	100–500	***	*	0	Moderate
Wellbutrin	bupropion	75–450	0	**	**	None
Wellbutrin SR	bupropion SR	100–400	0	**	**	None
Wellbutrin XL	bupropion XL	150–450	0	**	**	None

[1]Serzone no longer available by prescription; the generic, nefazodone is available by prescription.

* Minimal neurotransmission

** Moderate neurotransmission

*** Significant neurotransmission

TABLE 5.4 Monoamine Oxidase Inhibitors (MAOIs)

TRADE NAME	GENERIC NAME	TYPICAL DOSE (MG/DAY)	NEURO-TRANSMITTER 5-HT	NEURO-TRANSMITTER NE	NEURO-TRANSMITTER DA	LEVEL OF SEDATION
Marplan	isocarboxazid	10–40	**	**	**	Light
Nardil	phenelzine	30–90	**	**	**	Light
Parnate	tranylcypromine	20–60	**	**	**	Light

* Minimal neurotransmission

** Moderate neurotransmission

*** Significant neurotransmission

33

thinners like warfarin (Coumadin) and lessens the effectiveness of other heart medications like digoxin (Lanoxin). It may also interfere with protease inhibitors taken by HIV–AIDS patients. The active ingredient in St. John's wort is hypericum perforatum. Patients who are allergic to plant derivatives should not take St. John's wort, because they might break out in a rash or become seriously photophobic to it and experience severe burn when exposed to the sun. Patients should take hypericum perforatum in its liquid form, which assures that they get a true dose. Health food stores sell brands that may contain more inactive plant parts and less hypericum. St. John's wort should not be taken with other antidepressants, because it may potentiate their effects and cause serotonin syndrome.

Ginkgo biloba is a tree of Chinese origin. An extract from it is said to relieve mild depression and increase memory and concentration. While 60 mg/day of ginkgo biloba is typical for depression and mild memory concerns, as much as 120 mg/day has been used with Alzheimer's patients. Since it is said to have blood-thinning properties, ginkgo biloba should be used with caution by those taking blood-thinning medications. In our experience, it has not been as effective as antidepressants in the treatment of moderate to severe depression.

The hormone *dehydroepiandrosterone* or *DHEA* is normally secreted by the adrenal gland and is a precursor to testosterone and estrogen. Typically, adolescents have high levels of this substance, but the levels decrease with age. Some clinicians believe that when DHEA is taken orally, it reduces mild to moderate depression, causes weight loss, increases large muscle mass, and may increase sexual appetite. While these claims have yet to be fully proven, many practicing endocrinologists believe DHEA may increase the risk of certain types of cancer. Side effects are usually mild but may include oily skin, acne, irritability, and even psychosis.

S-adenosyl-L-methionine (SAM-e) is a substance that is endogenous to our body. It is essential to many biological processes such as cell methylation. The body converts SAM-e into the amino acid homocysteine, which accumulates and can cause depression, joint problems, and cancer. Homocysteine can be converted back into SAM-e by utilizing vitamins B_6, B_{12}, and folic acid. Research conducted in Italy has shown that depressed patients have much lower levels of SAM-e than nondepressed patients. Patients with poor diet typically make less SAM-e. It is now available as a synthesized substance and has been shown to be as effective as many prescription antidepressants for relieving depression. It is available as a prescription in many European countries. SAM-e may also be helpful in relieving joint pain and for cleansing the liver of other toxins. Researchers believe that SAM-e may increase the synthesis of serotonin and dopamine and aide in chemical communication between cells by potentiating the postsynaptic membrane.

LIGHT THERAPY FOR SEASONAL AFFECTIVE DISORDER (SAD)

Antidepressants have been shown to be helpful for patients with seasonal affective disorder; however, the use of light boxes is also effective. Therapists who treat patients living in colder, darker climates and suffering from seasonal depression might consider suggesting the use of a light box first unless the patient's depression worsens and he or she becomes suicidal. Several commercially produced lamps or boxes are available. They cost between $100 and $500. The light source should produce at least 10,000 lux of full-spectrum light. Patients will need to be directly exposed to the light for 30–60 minutes/day and sit approximately 10–12 inches from most light sources. Bulbs sold in hardware stores for use in overhead fixtures and in doorways may be esthetically pleasing, but they offer little in the form of treatment. Most quality lamps can be found by searching the Internet under seasonal affective disorders or full-spectrum lamps. In some cases, a letter from a physician or psychologist is required for the patient to purchase the lamp directly.

IMPORTANCE OF EXERCISE

Therapists should always encourage depressed patients to exercise. Not only does exercise lead to weight loss and increased levels of motivation, but it also helps to release important endorphins like phenylethylamine (PEA). The presence of PEA is associated with increased levels of endorphins and improvement in motivation, energy, and mood.

ELECTROCONVULSIVE THERAPY (ECT)

In some cases, patients with severe depression do not respond to antidepressants. If their depression worsens and includes suicidal ideation, they may be referred for ECT. Electroconvulsive therapy is given when the patient is anesthetized and paralyzed. Electrodes are placed on the scalp, usually on the nonspeech-dominant hemisphere to avoid later damage to verbal memories. Electricity is then administered, resulting in a seizure. No movement is noted because the patient is paralyzed or immobilized. Most patients receive three sessions per week for up to four weeks, or until improvement is noted. While excessive use of ECT may cause brain damage and memory loss, some researchers have noted that naloxone (Narcan), a drug that blocks opioid receptors, may reduce some of the adverse cognitive side effects of ECT (Prudic, et al. 1999). Some clinicians, especially those who treat elderly and medically ill patients, believe that the risks associated with ECT are equivalent or even preferable to many medications used to treat depression (Kelly & Zisselman, 2000).

For patients who may not be good candidates for ECT, new research into the use of transcranial magnetic stimulation or TMS to the prefrontal cortex, stimulation of the vagus nerve, and stimulation of other areas of the brain through deep brain stimulation may offer some relief (Triggs, et al., 1999; Klein, Kreinin, & Christyakov, et al., 2003).

PROCEDURAL STEPS FOR PATIENT TREATMENT

When a decision is made to use medication to treat a patient's depression, the therapist should follow a *treatment protocol* or procedural steps in both deciding on the appropriate medications and how to use them.

Step 1. Most prescribing professionals start with the easier medications first. These include the SSRIs such as fluoxetine (Prozac), citalopram (Celexa), sertraline (Zoloft), and so on. These medications have fewer side effects and interact with fewer other medications. In many cases, the patient is started on a low dose and titrated up. The patient must end up on a therapeutic dose of the medication to truly determine if the medication will be of use to him or her. Research suggests that too many patients are maintained on a too small dose of antidepressants, which is no better than no dose at all (Leon, Solomon, Mueller et al., 2003). (This is a common problem when primary care physicians write prescriptions.) If the patient has a satisfactory response and all symptoms appear to remit, the therapist should continue with psychotherapy and not increase the medication. The clinician may need to wait at least four to five weeks to determine the level of response.

Step 2. In some cases the patient has only a partial response to SSRIs, even when the dose is increased. Since SSRIs only affect the neurotransmitter serotonin, the patient's depression may be related to norepinephrine and/or dopamine. In such cases, additional medications aimed at the other neurotransmitters might need to be added or substituted. It is not unusual for such patients to be taking an SSRI like fluoxetine and also taking venlafaxine (Effexor) or bupropion (Wellbutrin). Polypharmacy is more complicated and should not be attempted by the patient's primary care physician. In addition, antidepressants can be augmented or "boosted" by adding a low dose of lithium for one or two weeks, or by adding a stimulant like methylphenidate (Ritalin). Buspirone (Buspar), a nonbenzodiazepine anxiety medication with antidepressant qualities, and folic acid may also boost the antidepressant response.

Step 3. If the patient appears to have psychotic features in addition to his or her depression, an appropriate neuroleptic or antipsychotic medication might need to be added to the regime. In rare cases, the patient may also have racing thoughts that interfere with his or her ability to relax. In these cases, neuroleptics may also be added to calm the thoughts and allow the patient to sleep better. Refer to Chapter 8 for further information on these medications.

Step 4. If the therapist and the prescriber have tried several drugs with no response, they should check with the patient to determine if he or she is using alcohol or other substances, taking the medication as directed, not taking the medication at all, and/or taking an unreported dietary supplement.

Step 5. The therapist should keep in mind that certain medications are contraindicated for certain types of patients. For patients with poor appetite or eating disorders, do not use bupropion as it may decrease appetite. For overweight patients, use mirtazepine (Remeron) and TCAs with caution, as they have been shown to cause an increase in weight and appetite. Patients with a history of seizure should not take bupropion because it lowers the seizure threshold. Nefazodone must be used with extra caution because it may cause liver failure in some patients. It is important to remember that MAOIs do not mix with other antidepressants and can cause a hypertensive crisis. It is imperative to wait at least two weeks after using an MAOI before starting another antidepressant because of potential drug interactions; the prescriber must wait two weeks after stopping another medication before trying MAOIs. There is one exception; the prescriber should wait five weeks after discontinuing fluoxetine before MAOIs are used.

Effective therapy includes *patient education*. As mentioned earlier, patients with dysthymia or minor depression typically are not placed on medication unless they are experiencing sleep difficulties, or the depression is seriously affecting their ability to function, which is true for patients who are experiencing serious complications to grief. For patients who are suffering from major depressive episodes and who are found to be good candidates for pharmacology, the therapist should inform them of the following five facts where appropriate:

1. Antidepressant medications take time to work. Typically a patient waits between one and four weeks before an antidepressant begins to work. Advise the patient to be patient! Some medications, like venlafaxine (Effexor) may begin to work within a couple of days, but this is the exception, not the rule.

2. Inform the patient about the types of side effects to expect from the medication he or she is taking. It is easy to remember the major side effects with antidepressants, as they all start with the letter S. The side effects include sexual, sedation, seizure, and stomach related symptoms. In most cases, these side effects are minimal and most of them disappear within a few days. Try not to spend too much time taking about side effects, because the patient may begin to fear the medication and refuse to take it. The following is a list of typical side effects and how best to resolve them.

- Dry mouth: increase water consumption, chew gum, use hard candy (avoid TCAs)
- Inability to orgasm: reduce dose of SSRI; switch to bupropion (Wellbutrin); add low dose mirtazepine (Remeron), bupropion, buspirone (Buspar), nefazodone (Serzone), or cyproheptadine; also, consider switching to duloxetine (Cymbalta)
- Forgetfulness: add bupropion, ginkgo biloba, or stimulant
- Insomnia: check for serotonin syndrome, add sedative-hypnotic, trazodone or nefazodone
- Sedation: avoid TCAs, paroxetine (Paxil), and nefazodone; use fluoxetine (Prozac), venlafaxine or bupropion
- Weight gain: avoid TCAs or mirtazepine, consider bupropion or other SSRIs
- Stomach upset: take with food, avoid SSRIs if GI upset is severe
- Headache: treat with acetaminophen (Tylenol) or aspirin if severe
- Hand tremors: reduce dose, add low-dose benzodiazepine

3. Remind the patient that he or she should never stop the medications abruptly. This may cause the patient to experience a type of withdrawal known as discontinuation syndrome, which is accompanied by severe flulike symptoms. If the patient is concerned about the medications, he or she needs to discuss the problem with the therapist and the prescribing professional. If a decision is made to stop a medication, it should be done gradually and under medical supervision. Watch for an increase in depression or suicidal ideation.

4. Pregnant patients should probably not take antidepressants (or any other medication) if they can help it. The clinician should consider antidepressant only if the patient is severely depressed and cannot function without them. Typically, antidepressants are most dangerous in the first trimester. Teratogenicity data and practice experience have indicated that SSRIs and bupropion are generally safer than other antidepressants. Lithium and antipsychotic medication should be avoided or only used under strict medical supervision. Breast-feeding mothers should consult their physician before they proceed.

5. Typically, antidepressants will relieve symptoms of depression and associated anxiety. Many patients today are concerned about taking drugs and will resist the therapist's recommendations. When working with a severely depressed patient for whom psychotherapy alone has not helped, the therapist must help the patient to see that medication may be a very important part of treatment. The therapist may find it helpful to use the analogy of vitamins for the person who is malnourished. Antidepressants allow the brain and neurotransmitters to work better leading to improved emotional functioning.

CHAPTER SIX

TREATMENT OF BIPOLAR DISORDER

This chapter reviews the types and causes of bipolar illness, as well as current information on treatment options for this population. Polypharmacy and family education will also be discussed.

Topics to be addressed include the following:

- Prevalence and types of bipolar illness
- Causes of bipolar disorder
- Counseling and psychotherapy
- Medications for bipolar disorders
- Treatment resistance and protocol
- Patient and family education

PREVALENCE AND TYPES OF BIPOLAR ILLNESS

Bipolar illness is a disorder of mood regulation characterized by cycling between high-highs or *mania* and low-lows or *depression*. Although effective treatments are available, three out of four patients will fail maintenance treatment within five years (Moller & Nasrallah, 2003). The lifetime prevalence of *bipolar disorder* is approximately 1 percent of the general population when a strict DSM-IV definition is used (Malhi, Mitchell, & Salim, 2003). When the broader term *bipolar spectrum disorders* is used, Grunze, Schlosser, and Walden (2000) report that the lifetime prevalence increases to 3 to 6 percent. Bipolar disorder usually begins with an index depressive episode about 50 percent of the time. The average age of onset of the first depressive episode is 18.7 years, and the first manic episode is 24.5 years. Unfortunately, the average age of the correct bipolar diagnosis is typically delayed until 33.5 years.

In contrast to unipolar depression, bipolar disorder is thought to originate endogenously but may be triggered by exogenous or environmental stimuli. Monozygotic twins have a 40 to 70 percent concordance rate, whereas dizygotic twins or first-degree relatives have only a 5 to 10 percent chance of inheriting the illness (Craddock

& Jones, 1999). The mainstay of treatment is therefore derived from a biological perspective, that is, medications. Psychosocial stressors may trigger the patient to *cycle* or may cause a more severe cycle. Although some environmental factors influence the disorder, it is commonly known that a genetic predisposition or vulnerability is necessary.

There are many different types of bipolar spectrum disorders. Bipolar Disorder Type I is a well-defined symptom cluster that may present as manic features, depressive features, or mixed-mood states. Bipolar Disorder Type II is similar but limited to hypomanic states only. In addition, cyclothymia is considered to be the milder form of the classic disease that is characterized by cycles between hypomania and low-level depression. Another useful term to know is *rapid cycling*, which is defined as the occurrence of four or more episodes of mania or depression in a 12-month period. The most common cause of rapid cycling is the uncritical use of antidepressant medications (Grunze, Schlosser & Walden, 2000).

When compared to unipolar depression, bipolar depression is associated with higher rates of suicide and psychosis. Primarily during the depressive cycle, approximately 10 to 20 percent of bipolar patients will complete suicide (Goodwin, 2002). According to Bowden (2001), psychotic symptoms occur in the context of bipolar Type I disorder about 50 to 90 percent of the time. Comorbidity commonly occurs in bipolar patients with anxiety disorders and substance abuse problems being the most prevalent. Cormorbidity will be covered more extensively in Chapter 13, Chemical Dependency and Co-Occuring Conditions.

CAUSES OF BIPOLAR DISORDER

When evaluating a bipolar patient, the psychiatric symptoms are only one component of a larger dynamic functioning person. While an exact cause of bipolar conditions is not well understood, it is theorized that the cause may be related to neurotransmitter dysregulation or possibly abnormal permeability of the postsynaptic membrane. The clinician needs to exclude medical issues that might cause or contribute to a patient's cycling mood disorder. The following is a list of diseases and disorders that have been associated with or known to exacerbate mania:

Brain tumors

Carcinoid syndrome

CNS syphilis

CNS trauma

Delirium (multiple etiologies)

Encephalitis (herpes and other viruses)

Huntington's disease

Influenza

Hyperthyroidism

Metabolic changes (electrolyte abnormalities)

Metastatic cancer

Multiple sclerosis

Parkinson's disease

Pellagra (deficiency of nicotinic acid)

Postpartum metabolic changes

Renal failure and hemodialysis

Stroke

Temporal lobe epilepsy

Vitamin B_{12} deficiency

Wilson's disease

Furthermore, many medications and other substances have been known to cause or worsen a patient's mania. These substances are often overlooked when a patient presents to medical providers. The following is a list of these medications and substances:

Antidepressants (pharmaceuticals and herbals)

Antihypertensive medications: captopril, hydralazine

Baclofen

Bromides

Bromocryptine

Cimetidine

Corticosteroids and other hormones: prednisone, testosterone

Cyclosporine

Disulfiram

Drugs of abuse: amphetamines, cocaine, ephedra, hallucinogens, PCP

Isoniazid

Levodopa

Opiates and opioids

Procarbazine

Procyclidine

Psychostimulants: dextroamphetamine, methylphenidate

Yohimbine

COUNSELING AND PSYCHOTHERAPY

After a thorough clinical assessment and medical evaluation, the therapist prepares an appropriate treatment plan for the patient. In addition to pharmacotherapy and possible hospitalization, the patient will most likely need psychotherapy when he or she has stabilized on medications. Remember that mild forms of unipolar depression may be treated with psychotherapy alone. However, pharmacotherapy is the cornerstone of treatment with psychotherapy playing a lesser role with bipolar mood disorder. Suicide assessment is still an important part of any evaluation. Bipolar patients have a higher risk of suicide because of their erratic and chaotic mood swings and behaviors.

One of the first steps a counselor or psychotherapist should address is basic family education regarding the illness. Most families have little understanding of the symptoms, behavioral management, causes, or treatments needed for the identified patient. Many educational resources are available through organizations such as the National Institute of Mental Health (NIMH), National Alliance for the Mentally Ill (NAMI), or Depression and Bipolar Support Alliance (formerly National Depressive and Manic Depressive Association). Family therapy should focus on establishing a safe environment, constructive communication, and solving problems together. The patient might benefit from individual psychotherapy to help him or her understand the illness, accept the diagnosis, and learn to manage the chronic nature of the disorder. Psychotherapists know that various forms of psychotherapy may be appropriate, including psychodynamic, cognitive-behavioral, or solution focused.

MEDICATIONS FOR BIPOLAR DISORDER

Psychopharmacology for bipolar disorder involves a class of medications known as *mood stabilizers*. The list of mood stabilizers consists of three broad categories, including lithium, anticonvulsants, and atypical antipsychotics. The choice of treatment options depends on whether the patient is in the manic, depressed, or mixed phase of the illness. These options will be discussed in more detail in the following sections.

Lithium

Lithium has been the gold standard for treating bipolar disorder since the early 1970s. Indications for lithium include treatment of acute mania and as maintenance therapy to prevent subsequent cycling. Furthermore, both manic and depressive phases of the bipolar cycle may be treated with lithium. Although lithium's mechanism of action is still unknown, Schatzberg, Cole, and DeBattista (1997) have found that there are multiple biochemical effects including the following:

- Increases synthesis of serotonin
- Enhances release of serotonin
- Increases rate of synthesis/excretion of norepinephrine in depressed patients
- Decreases rate of synthesis/excretion of norepinephrine in manic patients
- Blocks postsynaptic dopamine receptors' supersensitivity
- Has direct or indirect effect of G proteins that mediates balance of neurotransmitters
- Inhibitis enzymes in the phosphoinositide (PI) second messenger system that may affect receptor activity of many neurotransmitters

Since lithium acts as a salt in the body, lithium concentration is determined by the patient's body fluid status. Lithium is not metabolized in the liver and is excreted unchanged by the kidneys. Thus, when dehydration occurs, the kidneys may reabsorb more lithium, which might lead to toxicity. Because of the pharmacokinetics of lithium, the therapeutic level is close to the toxic level, thus, this medication has a low *therapeutic index* (refer to Chapter 3 for more explanation).

The most common side effects of lithium include increased thirst, increased urination, rash, tremor, dry mouth, increased appetite with weight gain, nausea, bloating, diarrhea, edema, and thyroid dysfunction. The side effects of the drug may be diminished by using divided doses throughout the day rather than one daily dose. In rare cases lithium toxicity may cause renal insufficiency or failure. Although this effect sounds terrible, lithium may be used with success when it is monitored appropriately by the prescribing professional.

Lithium is usually started at 300 mg/day and increased to a therapeutic dose of 600–1200 mg/day (see Table 6.1). Laboratory testing is usually done before initiating therapy and subsequently at regular intervals (about every six months) when the patient is stable. Therapeutic levels of lithium are usually in the range of 0.7–0.9 mEq/L while the toxic rage is typically 1.5 mEq/L or above.

Signs of lithium toxicity include ataxia, poor coordination, slurred speech, poor attention span, severe tremors, severe nausea/vomiting, lethargy, arrhythmias, hypotension, seizure, coma, and death. Lithium use in pregnancy has been contraindicated historically because of an association with congenital heart malformation. More recently, the risk is only rated as moderate (Viguera, Cohen, Baldessarini, Nonacs, 2002).

Anticonvulsants

In addition to lithium, there is another class of mood stabilizers known as anticonvulsants or antiseizure medications. Researchers believe that some of the anticonvulsants increase the concentration of GABA, the inhibitory neurotransmitter. By increasing inhibition, electrical activity is diminished and less neurotransmission occurs.

Valproate.   The most well-known medication in the anticonvulsant group is valproic acid or valproate (Depakote). Unlike lithium, valproate may be more useful in patients with rapid cycling, atypical features, or mixed-mood states. Valproate has been FDA approved for treatment of acute mania and as an adjunctive therapy with other agents. The most common side effects of valproate include nausea, diarrhea, hair loss, rash, weight gain, and tremor. Laboratory testing is required with valproate to evaluate the serum concentration, complete blood count, and liver function tests. Although the therapeutic index is wider when compared to lithium, valproate serum concentrations of 150 micrograms/ml or greater only lead to more side effects without any improved clinical response. Valproate is not used during pregnancy because of the high risk of neural tube defects, for example, spina bifida and anencephaly.

Carbamazepine.   Another anticonvulsant that has widespread use as a mood stabilizer is carbamazepine (Tegretol). Although this medication has been extensively

TABLE 6.1 Mood Stabilizers

TRADE NAME	GENERIC NAME	TYPICAL DOSE (MG/DAY)	PROPOSED MECHANISM OF ACTION
Lithobid, Eskalith CR	lithium carbonate or lithium citrate	600–1200	Enhances serotonin, increases or decreases norepinephrine, blocks dopamine receptors' supersensitivity, alters second messengers
Depakote, Depakote ER	valproate or valproic acid	500–2000	Inhibition of sodium and/or calcium channels, increases GABA, releases glutamate
Tegretol, Tegretol XR, Carbatrol	carbamazepine	600–1200	Inhibition of sodium channels
Lamictal	lamotrigine	200–400	Inhibition of sodium channels, presynaptic modulation of glutamate release
Neurontin	gabapentin	300–3600	Enhances GABA
Topamax	topiramate	100–500	Increases GABA, blocks glutamate receptors
Gabitril	tiagabine	8–16	Increases GABA
Zonegran	zonisamide	200–400	Inhibition of sodium and/or calcium channels, facilitates dopaminergic and serotonergic neurotransmission
Trileptal	oxcarbazepine	600–1200	Inhibition of sodium channels, modulation of calcium channels
Klonopin	clonazepam	2–6	Increases GABA
Zyprexa, Zyprexa Zydis	olanzepine	10–30	Dopamine type 2 and serotonin type 2 antagonism
Symbyax	fluoxetine/ olanzepine	6–12/ 25–50	Inhibition of serotonin reuptake/ dopamine type 2 and serotonin type 2 antagonism
Risperdal, Risperdal M-tab	risperidone	2–6	Dopamine type 2 and serotonin type 2 antagonism
Seroquel	quetiapine	400–600	Dopamine type 2 and serotonin type 2 antagonism
Geodon	ziprasidone	80–160	Dopamine type 2 and serotonin type 2 antagonism
Abilify	aripiprazole	15–30	Partial agonism at dopamine type 2 and serotonin type 1A, serotonin type 2A antagonism
Clozaril	clozapine	300–600	Low dopamine type 2 antagonism, high dopamine type 1 and type 4 antagonism, high serotonin type 2 antagonism
Verelan PM, Covera-HS, Ispotin SR	verapamil	200–400	Calcium channel blocker

studied, it does not have FDA approval for use as a mood stabilizer. The most common side effects of carbamazepine include rash, fatigue, nausea, dizziness, and sedation. As with lithium and valproate, carbamazepine requires laboratory monitoring because of the possibility of agranulocytosis (decreased white blood cell count) and aplastic anemia (decreased production of all blood cells); however, both of these effects are rare. Drug interactions with carbamazepine may be more problematic, and the prescribing professional should be aware of the pitfalls. As with valproate, the use of carbamazeprine in pregnancy carries a high risk of multiple fetal anomalies.

Lamotrigine.   Lamotrigine (Lamictal) is a newer generation of anticonvulsants that obtained FDA approval in 2003 for maintenance treatment of bipolar disorder. This medication appears to be superior to the other mood stabilizers for bipolar depression. The most important side effect to remember about lamotrigine is the potential for a *toxic rash* (Stevens-Johnson syndrome). Other common side effects include headache, dizziness, and sedation. The risk of this medication in pregnancy is virtually unknown.

Gabapentin.   Gabapentin (Neurontin) is also used in the treatment of bipolar disorder primarily as an adjunctive treatment. This drug has been used clinically and has some research basis but has not been approved by the FDA for use in bipolar disorder. The most common side effects of gabapentin include sedation, tremors, nausea, dizziness, and weight gain. The use of gabapentin during pregnancy is not recommended.

Topiramate.   Topiramate (Topamax) might be another useful alternative, but like gabapentin, it does not have the FDA indication. This drug may have one major advantage over the others: It does not cause weight gain. The most common side effects of topiramate include weight loss, sedation, cognitive dulling, fatigue, headache, and paresthesias (numbness in extremities). The use of topiramate during pregnancy is not recommended.

Other Anticonvulsant Medications.   A few other anticonvulsant mood stabilizers worth mentioning include tiagabine (Gabitril) and zonisamide (Zonegran). They are similar to the other medications mentioned that are being researched for use in bipolar disorder. Oxcarbazepine (Trileptal) is a medication similar to carbamazepine but does not carry the risk of agranulocytosis or aplastic anemia. Further investigation of oxcarbazepine is needed to fully confirm or deny its usefulness in bipolar disorder. Clonazepam (Klonopin) is another anticonvulsant medication, which happens to be a benzodiazepine. It is used primarily as an adjunctive treatment in patients who do not have a history of chemical dependency problems.

Atypical Antipsychotic Medications

In addition to lithium and the anticonvulsants, the final category of mood stabilizers are the atypical antipsychotic medications.

Olanzepine (Zyprexa).   The first antipsychotic mediation to receive FDA approval for acute mania was olanzepine. When a patient presents with mania and psychosis, olanzepine is the drug of choice, because it functions both as a mood stabilizer and an antipsychotic. Olanzepine has received FDA approval for acute monotherapy treatment, maintenance monotherapy treatment, and combination treatment for bipolar disorder. The medication also comes in an alternative form, Zyprexa Zydis (orally disintegrating tablet), which is used in hospital settings where compliance is called into question. The most common side effects of olanzepine include sedation, weight gain, constipation, dry mouth, dizziness, orthostatic hypotension, and weakness. When a patient takes olanzepine, laboratory monitoring of glucose, lipids, and liver functions are recommended because of the likelihood of the drug causing diabetes, hypercholesterolemia, and liver dysfunction. The use of olanzepine in pregnancy is not recommended.

Symbyax.   Another medication approved by the FDA, specifically for the depressive phase of bipolar disorder is known as Symbyax. This medication is a combination of fluoxetine (Prozac) and olanzepine. More information about the individual medications can be found in Chapters 5 and 8.

Risperidone.   Another antipsychotic medication that has mood stabilizing properties is risperidone (Risperdal). It has been approved by the FDA as monotherapy or adjunctive therapy for treatment of acute manic or mixed episodes. As with Zyprexa Zydis, Risperdal has an orally disintegrating tablet called Risperdal M-tab. The most common side effects include restlessness, insomnia, constipation, and dizziness. Recommendations for laboratory monitoring are basically the same as with olanzepine. Risperidone use during pregnancy carries significant risk and is not recommended.

Quetiapine.   Another antipsychotic medication, quetiapine (Seroquel), may be useful with acute mania. It is currently approved by the FDA for acute mania either as monotherapy or adjunctive therapy. Quetiapine's side effects include sedation, dizziness, constipation, and dry mouth. As with the other atypical antipsychotic medications, laboratory monitoring of blood sugar and lipids is recommended when using quetiapine. It is not recommended during pregnancy.

Ziprasidone.   Ziprasidone (Geodon) is another option available for acute mania, with or without psychosis. As of 2005, the drug is not approved for use in bipolar disorder and is only indicated for treating schizophrenia. Compared with the other atypical agents, ziprasidone has a greater capacity to cause QT prolongation on EKG, which is associated with a potentially fatal arrhythmia. The most common side effects include somnolence, dizziness, rash, anxiety, and nausea. Laboratory monitoring of glucose, lipids, and liver functions is recommended. Ziprasidone use during pregnancy is not recommended unless potential benefit to the mother outweighs potential risks to the fetus.

Aripiprazole.   The newest atypical antipsychotic available is aripiprazole (Abilify). This medication is clinically effective as a mood stabilizer also. In late 2004, the FDA approved Abilify for use in acute manic or mixed episodes. The most common side effects of aripiprazole include headache, nausea, insomnia, and somnolence. Laboratory monitoring is again necessary. As with other newer medications, aripiprazole is not recommended during pregnancy.

Clozapine.   The last atypical antipsychotic medication that is worth noting is clozapine (Clozaril). Although this medication is only approved for treatment-resistant schizophrenia, clozapine has been used for the last decade to manage severe mania in some circumstances. This drug is only used in select cases, because it may have very severe side effects including agranulocytosis and seizures. Clozapine requires weekly monitoring of the white blood cell (WBC) count for the first six months, then every other week while the patient remains on the drug. Other common side effects include weight gain, sedation, headache, orthostatic hypotension, constipation, salivation, tachycardia (increased heart rate), and myocarditis (inflammation of the heart). Clozapine is definitely an effective medication but requires more intense monitoring by the prescribing professional. Interestingly, clozapine is not known to be teratogenic and may be used in pregnancy if the benefits outweigh the risks. Clozapine comes in an orally disintegrating tablet form known as Fazaclo.

Typical Antipsychotic Medications

As opposed to *atypical* antipsychotic medications, a multitude of other *typical* antipsychotic medications are used adjunctively with other mood stabilizers. Haloperidol (Haldol), fluphenazine (Prolixin), trifluoperazine (Stelazine), thioridazine (Mellaril), and chlorpromazine (Thorazine) are a few of the most well-known agents. These medications are used primarily for acute agitation while the patient is hospitalized. Haloperidol and some of the other medications may be given intramuscularly or by mouth depending on the acuity of the situation. Although this class may cause major side effects including extrapyramidal symptoms, typical antipsychotics are used for behavioral management only in the short term (less than one week). More information about these medications may be found in Chapter 8, Treatment of Psychotic Disorders.

Other Medications

In addition to the medications already discussed, some other options are worth mentioning. Verapamil is a calcium-channel blocker that is primarily used in the treatment of hypertension, angina, and supraventricular arrhythmias. A small number of open trials suggest that the drug has antimanic properties. One randomized, double-blind, placebo-controlled study did not show any antimanic effect (Bowden, 2001).

Benzodiazepines are useful medications that may be used adjunctively with other mood stabilizers. For example, lorazepam (Ativan) is commonly given to manic patients early in their treatment to decrease agitation, which helps with behavioral management, until the primary mood stabilizer becomes effective. Finally, some researchers believe that omega-3 fatty acids may be helpful when taken in combination with lithium as compared to lithium alone. Although omega-3 fatty acids may have other health benefits, their use in bipolar disorder is still being debated.

ELECTROCONVULSIVE THERAPY (ECT)

In some severe manic patients, who are unresponsive to medications, a course of electroconvulsive therapy (ECT) is appropriate. During the depressed phase of the illness with suicidality present, ECT may be an option for a rapid response. As with any treatment option, the benefits of ECT must be weighed against the risks before proceeding. See the discussion in Chapter 5 for more information.

TREATMENT RESISTANCE AND PROTOCOL

Mania Treatment Protocol

As with depression, bipolar disorder requires a logical approach to medication decision making, depending on the phase of the bipolar cycle.

Step 1. The first place to start is with FDA approved medications for treatment of acute mania. For example, lithium or valproate would be first-line agents. If psychotic symptoms are present, olanzepine or another atypical antipsychotic might also be appropriate. The acutely manic patient is typically hospitalized during this phase of treatment. As noted earlier, a therapeutic dose or level of a particular medication is necessary. These medications need from five to fifteen days in a patient's system before a response may be evaluated.

Step 2. If the first drug trial fails or the patient is unable to tolerate the secondary side effects, an alternative is chosen. For example, if the patient started with lithium first, he or she may then be switched to valproate, or vice versa.

Step 3. If monotherapy fails, the next step would be a two-drug combination. Lithium plus an anticonvulsant, two anticonvulsants, or either of the previous with an atypical antipsychotic would be reasonable choices. If the patient fails to respond or only partially responds, a different two-drug combination therapy would be indicated. Most experts recommend continuing the various two-drug combinations until all are exhausted or the patient responds.

Step 4. If the two-drug combinations fail, the next step would be a triple-drug combination. The most common formula would include one drug from each of the main categories: lithium, an anticonvulsant, and an atypical antipsychotic. For the patient who gets to this level of difficulty, ECT or clozapine would also be appropriate options to consider. Remember that benzodiazepines and typical antipsychotics are used as adjunctive therapies throughout each step that is presented here.

Step 5. If the patient is not responding to the treatment plan, the clinician should take a step back and reassess the diagnosis, comorbid medical conditions, compliance issues, and/or substance-abuse issues. Clinicians must stay alert to changes in the patient's illness and must reassess the situation at every step along the way.

Depression Treatment Protocol

In addition to the mania protocol, the depressive phase of bipolar disorder requires the prescriber to consider some alternative issues.

Step 1. The primary medication to treat bipolar disorder, regardless of phase, is a mood stabilizer. When a patient is in the depressive phase, the mood stabilizer should be optimized first, usually by increasing the dosage. For example, lithium therapy should be increased to obtain a serum concentration of 0.7–0.9 mEq/L.

Step 2. The addition of an antidepressant such as an SSRI or bupropion would be the next choice. Remember that each medication must be given at an adequate dose and for an appropriate amount of time to see if the patient will respond. Another option would be to add lamotrigine rather than to add an antidepressant. As mentioned earlier, lamotrigine has a specific niche for bipolar depression. The prescriber must be cautious when using lamotrigine with valproate because of the significantly elevated risk for the toxic rash.

Step 3. If the patient fails to respond to the previous steps, a combination of two antidepressants would be used with the mood stabilizer. For example, venlafaxine or nefazodone are other antidepressants that might be added to an SSRI or bupropion. Lamotrigine may be added once again to another antidepressant at this stage in order to obtain a response.

Step 4. The next choice in this process would include adding an atypical antipsychotic medication or a monoamine oxidase inhibitor (MAOI). Further steps beyond this include using ECT, thyroid hormones, typical antipsychotics, tricyclic antidepressants, hormones, omega-3 fatty acids, psychostimulants, and so on.

Treatment Protocol for Mixed-Mood States

Although there may be some similarities with the mania protocol, the treatment of mixed-mood states needs to be further explained.

Step 1. Atypical forms of bipolar disorder respond preferentially to anticonvulsants or atypical antipsychotics rather than to lithium. For example, valproate or olanzepine would be first-line treatments. As noted in the other protocols, the prescriber may need to optimize the dose in order to achieve the maximum response.

Step 2. If monotherapy with one medication fails, then monotherapy with the other agent would be appropriate. For example, valproate would be given if olanzepine was unsuccessful, or vice versa.

Step 3. As noted in the mania protocol, two-drug combinations would reasonably be followed by triple-drug combinations, and so on. The most important factor to consider is keeping a logical approach to this complex behavioral disorder. In other words, keep the treatment plan simple.

PATIENT AND FAMILY EDUCATION

Patient Education

The counselor or psychotherapist must assess the patient's level of understanding for his or her illness and try to fill in the gaps when necessary. The first step in this process is basic patient education about the natural history, symptoms, comorbidities, and various treatments of bipolar disorder. The best way for the patient to learn about his or her own illness is by reading and by talking to others who have the same problems. Support groups give patients an opportunity to learn from others and to help normalize their experiences. Compliance with medications is an enormous problem with bipolar patients, because they will often miss the euphoric mania. In fact, lithium is known to be less effective the more it is started and stopped for whatever reasons.

Comorbid alcohol or drug abuse is also common with bipolar patients and should be assessed routinely. It is not uncommon for a patient to minimize his or her use of "recreational" methamphetamine, which may be complicating the patient's response or lack thereof to the medications. Another example is the patient who forgets to inform the prescriber about drinking one or two martinis before or during dinner, which is likely contributing to the patient's symptomatology. The clinician should keep in mind that these types of patients have little concept of balance in their life, because they live between the extremes.

Family Education

As noted previously, family education is very important because the patient's life has a context that needs to be understood by family members. Remember that the manic phase of the illness, primarily the euphoria, feels really great to the patient. The clinician can help the family to understand that the patient may not want to lose this feeling. Family members may be helpful in monitoring the patient's compliance with medications and appointments. Any competent clinician would enlist the patient's family to assess symptomatology, compliance issues, and be involved in implementing the treatment plan. Moreover, the family will be the clinician's eyes and ears while the patient is at home.

The psychotherapist can be helpful by referring family members for their own individual treatment when they are having difficulty coping with the patient's behaviors. Although the most experienced clinician may be overwhelmed at times by the patient's bipolar illness, keep in mind that the family assists the patient on a daily basis to manage the symptoms.

TREATMENT OF ANXIETY DISORDERS

This chapter explores the symptoms associated with anxiety conditions, the general concept of anxiety, and its role in behavior. A biological explanation for panic states is explored along with the various treatment options and cautions.

Topics to be addressed include the following:

- Symptoms and causes of anxiety disorders
- Panic disorder with or without agoraphobia
- Generalized anxiety disorder
- Posttraumatic stress disorder
- Obsessive-compulsive disorder
- Adjustment disorders and other phobic conditions
- Social anxiety disorder
- Treatment reminders and cautions

SYMPTOMS AND CAUSES OF ANXIETY DISORDERS

Second only to depression and alcohol abuse, anxiety disorders are commonly presented in both mental health and medical/fact surgical settings. A well-known fact is that anxious patients overly use medical services (Lindesay, 1991). The pathophysiology of most anxiety disorders is rather complex and most likely linked to abnormal regulation of neurotransmitters such as serotonin, GABA, and glutamate. Additionally, a strong comorbidity exists among anxiety disorders, and while they often have similar symptoms, the manifestation or presentation might be different. Since the symptoms of most anxiety disorders are similar, the pharmacological treatment is the same (Bourin and Lambert, 2002).

Anxiety disorders typically include the following symptoms in various forms and intensity: trembling, general nervousness or tension, shortness of breath, diarrhea, hot flashes, feelings of depersonalization, worry, agitation, initial insomnia, poor concentration, tingling, sweating, rapid heartbeat (tachycardia), frequent urination, and dizziness. In assessing these symptoms, the therapist needs to determine the intensity, duration, and quality of these symptoms. This information will help the therapist make the proper diagnosis and treatment.

Anxiety symptoms may result from many other physical conditions, so it is important to rule-out any of the following conditions:

Adrenal tumor	Hypoglycemia
Alcoholism or other substance abuse	Hyperthyroidism
Angina	Mitral valve prolapse
Cardiac arrhythmia or other cardiovascular problem	Parathyroid disease
	Postconcussion syndrome
Chronic sinus conditions	Premenstrual syndrome (PMS)
Cushing's disease	Seizure disorders
Delirium	

It is also important to remember that many substances or drugs may cause or exacerbate anxiety. These include amphetamines and other stimulants, diet medications and other appetite suppressants, certain asthma medications, decongestants, cocaine, caffeine, and steroids. Withdrawal from antidepressants, anxiolytics, and other substances of abuse may cause anxiety also.

Once a medical or substance etiology has been ruled out, the therapist needs to determine the type and nature of the anxiety and a likely diagnosis. Anxiety disorders are now categorized as follows:

Panic disorder or PD (with or without agoraphobia)

Agoraphobia with or without panic disorder

Generalized anxiety disorder or GAD

Posttraumatic stress disorder or PTSD

Obsessive-compulsive disorder or OCD

Social anxiety disorder

Adjustment disorder with anxious mood

Simple phobias

Treatment and choice of medication depends on the type and severity of the anxiety disorder. Research has consistently demonstrated that anxiety disorders respond well to psychotherapy and that relaxation, cognitive therapy, and cognitive-behavioral therapy work best (Bourin and Lambert, 2002; Gorman, 2002). Further, Gorman maintains that the combination of therapy and medication offers the best prognosis for resistance to relapse of symptoms. With this in mind, we will address each disorder mentioned above with the most efficacious approach based on research and our experience.

PANIC DISORDER WITH OR WITHOUT AGORAPHOBIA

Many patients present to a therapist with complaints of anxiety and believe that they have panic disorder. Patients often confuse periods of uncomfortable anxiety with actual panic attacks. However, for those patients who experience four or more intense attacks within a 1-month period, panic disorder is a seriously debilitating condition.

What exactly is happening in the panic disordered patient? Anxiety is caused when the brain perceives a threat of danger. In reaction to the fight-or-flight response, the limbic system goes on red alert. The body responds to a series of physiological reactions: the limbic system sends signals to the hypothalamus and the locus ceruleus; they in turn send signals to the pituitary, the thyroid, and the adrenal cortex. As a result, various hormones such as cortisol and adrenaline are produced, readying the body for attack; but with panic disorder, it is a false alarm. Panic disorder often runs in families, and the cause appears to be biological in nature. A dysregulation of the limbic system, serotonin depletion, excessive glutamate, and insufficient amounts of GABA may all be to blame. Panic can be induced in patients with panic disorder by injecting them with either lactic acid (a by-product of muscular activity) or cholecystokinin (CCK), which is a peptide produced by cells in the duodenum and in the brain. When large amounts of cortisol and adrenaline are produced, the patient is in a constant or chronic state of arousal. The effects of stress on the body cause these hormones to suppress immune functions and increase blood pressure. These chronic conditions have been linked to other medical illnesses, cardiac problems, and cancer.

On the surface of about 40 percent of nerve cells in the brain, including the locus ceruleus, are tiny gateways or receptor sites called *chloride-ion channels*. Chloride ions, which have a slightly negative charge, are found in the fluid surrounding each cell. The ion channel can be activated or opened when stimulated by the naturally occurring neurotransmitter GABA. As the channel opens, the chloride ions are drawn in. When the cell is infused with negative ions, the cell hyperpolarizes or relaxes. This causes a calming effect of the locus ceruleus. Benzodiazepines also bind at the chloride-ion channels causing a calming effect. This effect is also true for alcohol. (See Figure 7.1.)

The treatment for panic disorder involves three stages: (1) stop the panic, (2) regulate the limbic system with drugs that increase serotonin, and (3) provide appropriate psychotherapy to educate the patient and reduce anticipatory anxiety or self-defeating behaviors.

Stage 1. In this stage the therapist sees that the patient is experiencing intense anxiety and needs immediate relief. Many patients with panic disorder use or abuse alcohol, which binds with the chloride-ion channel to control their symptoms. Unfortunately as tolerance is experienced, the amount of alcohol is increased, resulting in addiction for many patients.

Benzodiazepines are the drugs of choice for quick relief of panic symptoms. Alprazolam (Xanax), lorazepam (Ativan), and oxazepam (Serax) offer the fastest relief based on their short half-lives (see Table 7.1). For many patients with panic disorder, the treatment ends here.

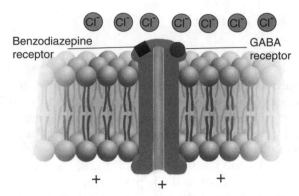

Phase 1: Choride ion channel closed (patient anxious)

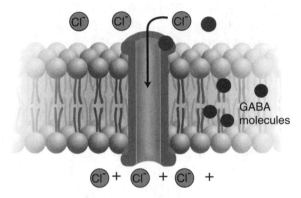

Phase 2: GABA binds to receptors: Channel begins to open

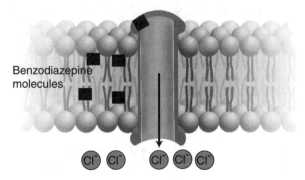

Phase 3: Benzodiazepine binds to receptors: Channel fully opens (patient relaxed)

FIGURE 7.1   Three Phases of the Chloride-Ion Channel

Primary care physicians often provide benzodiazepines to patients with panic disorder and forget to follow-up with them. These patients assume that since they are no longer panicking, they must be okay. Although the patients are no longer in a state of anxiety or having panic attacks, the use of benzodiazepines for panic disorder has only relieved the symptoms, but the cause remains.

TABLE 7.1   Various Medications Used in Anxiety Disorders

TRADE NAME	GENERIC NAME	TYPICAL DOSE (MG/DAY)	MEDICATION CLASS	USES
Ambien	zolpidem	5–10	Sedative-hypnotic	Sleep aid
Ativan	lorazepam	1–6	Benzodiazepine	PD, seizure, anxiety NOS
Buspar	buspirone	5–40	Nonbenzodiazepine	GAD, depression, anxiety NOS
Catapres	clonidine	0.1–0.3	Central alpha agonist	Hypertension, social anxiety disorder
Centrax	prazepam	20–60	Benzodiazepine	PD, anxiety NOS
Dalmane	flurazepam	15–30	Sedative-hypnotic	Sleep aid
Doral	quazepam	7.5–15	Sedative hypnotic	Sleep aid
Halcion	triazolam	0.25–0.50	Sedative-hypnotic	Sleep aid
Inderal	propranolol	20–80	Nonselective beta-blocker	Hypertension, social anxiety disorder
Klonopin	clonazepam	0.5–4	Benzodiazepine	PD, seizure, sleep aid, mood stabilizer
Librium	chlordiazepoxide	15–100	Benzodiazepine	Anxiety NOS, muscle relaxation
Lunesta	eszopiclone	1–3	Sedative-hypnotic	Sleep aid
Prosom	estazolam	2–4	Sedative-hypnotic	Sleep aid
Restoril	temazepam	15–30	Sedative-hypnotic	Sleep aid
Serax	oxazepam	30–120	Benzodiazepine	Anxiety NOS
Sonata	zaleplon	5–10	Sedative-hypnotic	Sleep aid
Tranxene	clorazepate	15–60	Benzodiazepine	Anxiety NOS
Valium	diazepam	5–40	Benzodiazepine	Seizure, anxiety NOS, muscle relaxation
Xanax	alprazolam	0.25–4	Benzodiazepine	PD, anxiety NOS

Generalized panic disorder (GAD), Panic disorder (PD), Not otherwise specified (NOS)

Stage 2. In this stage the therapist initiates antidepressant therapy. Once panic has been controlled with benzodiazepines, the use of various antidepressants will increase serotonin and help to regulate the limbic system. While some of the older tricyclics like imipramine, nortriptyline, and amitriptyline are used, the newer SSRIs offer better relief with fewer side effects. MAOIs will work as well, but dietary restrictions result in poor compliance for panic patients (see Chapter 5).

Stage 3. In this stage the therapist provides cognitive-behavioral treatment for patients with panic disorder. These patients must learn how to manage their anxiety without developing avoidance behaviors that are caused by experiencing panic attacks in places such as shopping malls. This *anticipatory anxiety* is actually more debilitating than panic itself. For patients with panic disorder and agoraphobia, or agoraphobia without panic disorder, the use of in vivo or real-life techniques are helpful. Encouraging patients to take walks outside of the home with the therapist and/or other treatment staff reduces isolation and discourages additional phobias from developing (Sinacola, 1997). For many patients with panic disorder, fears tend to compound the longer they go untreated. It is best to address fears early in therapy. As expected, many patients will be reluctant at first and may complain of increased levels of arousal until new relaxation and other therapeutic methods are understood and practiced.

With panic disorder it is very important for the therapist to address all three stages. Once the therapist determines that a patient truly has the condition, benzodiazepines should be started. The therapist should inquire about any history of substance abuse, because these patients often enjoy the "high" they get from benzodiazepines and may abuse them. It is worth noting here that the longer-acting benzodiazepines like clonazepam (Klonopin) are less likely to be abused than alprazolam (Xanax) or lorazepam (Ativan). The prescriber must include an appropriate antidepressant along with the benzodiazepine. The benzodiazepine will control panic, and within one to two weeks the antidepressant will begin to work. At this time, the benzodiazepine should be gradually withdrawn. It is crucial not to withdraw the benzodiazepine too quickly, as this may cause panic to return. Typically, withdrawing the benzodiazepines over a 2–3 weeks period is effective unless the patient has been taking the medication for a long period of time and the dose is high. The antidepressant should maintain patients if they are not abusing alcohol or other drugs. Psychotherapy may be attempted at any time during this process once the patient is calm enough to focus and concentrate in the session.

GENERALIZED ANXIETY DISORDER

Many practicing clinicians believe that generalized anxiety disorder or GAD is a behavioral condition and should not be treated with medication. Further, some researchers believe that GAD is more closely related to depression than to anxiety (Sheehan, 1999). Sheehan (1999) also found that people with GAD also utilized medical services more than those without the diagnosis.

Most patients with GAD respond well to a combination of medication and psychotherapy (Sheehan, 2002). Cognitive therapy is helpful as a form of psychoeducation that allows patients to see patterns in their perceptions of issues and the behaviors or actions that follow. While benzodiazepines have been used to treat GAD in the past, this use is not the best approach, because it does not teach patients to manage their condition.

Typically, the best medications for GAD include venlafaxine (Effexor), buspirone (Buspar), and most of the SSRIs such as fluoxetine (Prozac) and paroxetine (Paxil). Buspirone is a nonbenzodiazepine, antianxiety drug that has properties more similar to an antidepressant. As mentioned in Chapter 5, buspirone may alleviate depression for the anxious patient with co-occurring mood concerns. Unlike benzodiazepines, buspirone and the other antidepressants may take three to four weeks before they take effect. Patients need to be informed of this fact and they must be patient. Patients also need to be told that these medications should be taken as directed and not only as needed. If the patient is concerned about sedation, fluoxetine, venlafaxine, sertraline (Zoloft), citalopram (Celexa), and escitalopram (Lexapro) may be better choices. If the patient has serious trouble relaxing, buspirone or paroxetine may be better because they have a more relaxing and calming effect.

For many patients with GAD, initial insomnia is a problem. Sleep aids may be helpful for the short term, but many of them such as the newer drugs zolpidem (Ambien) and zaleplon (Sonata) may be habit forming in the long term. It is probably better to begin the antidepressant therapy and wait a week or two to see if sleep improves. If the patient is persistent, the clinician could recommend a low dose of a sedative-hypnotic. For example, 5–10 mg of zolpidem at bedtime for only one week reduces the likelihood of dependence. If the patient is concerned about taking prescription sleep aids, the clinician could recommend over-the-counter diphenhydramine (Benadryl) at 25–50 mg before bedtime. For patients with severe agitation and racing thoughts at bedtime, gabapentin (Neurontin) or an atypical neuroleptic may be needed (see Chapters 5 and 6, and Table 7.1).

POSTTRAUMATIC STRESS DISORDER

Historically, benzodiazepines and neuroleptics have been used to treat patients with posttraumatic stress disorder (PTSD), especially when they demonstrate psychotic-type behaviors (Albucher and Liberzon, 2002). Today, considering reported overall efficacy and side-effect profiles, clinicians have found much success with SSRIs. In some cases, mood stabilizers like lamotrigine (Lamictal) and atypical neuroleptics (i.e., risperidone or olanzepine) might be needed if the patient becomes agitated, combative, or psychotic. Psychotherapy is a very important part of the treatment for PTSD. Patients may need to slowly expose themselves to the event or events that contributed to the condition. Like bipolar patients, PTSD patients typically abuse substances in an attempt to dull the pain and anxiety. Detoxification may be needed first to ensure successful use of psychotropic medications. While any antidepressant would be helpful, SSRIs like paroxetine and sertraline have been approved for such use.

OBSESSIVE-COMPULSIVE DISORDER

Obsessive-compulsive disorder (OCD) is more of a worldwide health problem than once thought. Approximately 3 percent of the population suffers from OCD with typical onset in patients in their twenties. (Jenike, 2001). Psychotherapy alone has not been shown to be very effective; behavioral and cognitive-behavioral treatments along with medication offer the best possibilities.

The cause of OCD remains unknown, but a familial link might exist since patients with OCD typically have a close relative who has OCD or OCD co-occurring with a tic disorder. The most likely cause of OCD is dysfunction in one or more of several segregated corticostriatal pathways. According to Jenike (2001), OCD seems to involve subtle structural abnormalities in the caudate nucleus, as well as functional dysregulation of neural circuits of the orbital frontal cortex, cingulate cortex, and the caudate nucleus. Some reseachers believe that childhood infections may have contributed to the development of OCD (Insel, 1992). In any case, serotonergic systems have been implicated.

The treatment of choice for OCD involves, the use of SSRIs. While the tricyclic clomipramine (Anafranil) has been used, sedation and anticholinergic side effects are troublesome. SSRIs affect serotonin levels and typically relieve symptoms. It is important to remember that the doses used for depression and other anxiety disorders might not be high enough for the OCD patient. Therefore, a dose of 60–80 mg of fluoxetine (Prozac) or 200–300mg of fluvoxamine (Luvox) may be needed for OCD relief (see Chapter 5 and Table 7.1). In some cases the obsessions are severely intrusive, and the patient may complain of racing thoughts and insomnia. Low-dose, atypical neuroleptics such as risperidone (Risperdal) could be added along with a sleep aid if needed.

SOCIAL ANXIETY DISORDER

Social anxiety disorder or social phobia is a common presenting issue in private practices and public clinics. In such cases the therapist needs to determine that the patient has never had a history of panic disorder. Many professionals believe that social anxiety should be treated with psychotherapy alone and medications should not be used; however, several medications have been found to be useful (Davidson, 2003). Many patients with social anxiety have found that alcohol relieves their symptoms, but they demonstrate obvious alcohol dysfunction in social situations. This dysfunction may lead to social or occupational problems, or worse, alcohol dependence. Typically, primary care physicians offer benzodiazepines to socially phobic patients. While these drugs may lessen patients' fears a bit, they do not afford patients an opportunity to understand their fears and subsequent behaviors.

The use of SSRIs and MAOIs offers the best results for social anxiety patients. Tricyclics, benzodiazepines, and buspirone (Buspar) offer little benefit in the long run. In some cases when the patient reports only situational anxiety, for example, when he or she has to speak publicly, the use of beta-blockers like propranolol (Inderal) or clonidine (Catapres), an alpha agonist, might prove helpful. In these cases the patient may take the medication an hour before the speech and notice less sweating, heart palpitations, and general anxiety without the need to take medication on an ongoing basis.

Psychotherapy, especially behaviorally based treatments, are helpful in allowing the patient an opportunity to see the connection between environments and the fears they produce. Cognitive rehearsal and role plays may assist the patient in a more lasting recovery.

ADJUSTMENT DISORDERS AND OTHER PHOBIC CONDITIONS

When a patient presents with anxiety and sleep disturbance related to a stressful event, the clinician must rule out PTSD, GAD, or another long-standing anxiety disorder. If the patient appears to have no history of an anxiety disorder and he or she seems to be aware of the stressor that might be responsible, counseling and psychotherapy is recommended. In most cases the symptoms will remit within six months. A sleep aide could be used for a short period of time if the patient complains of ongoing problems with insomnia. If the patient appears to have significant anxiety, a low-dose SSRI could be used for four to six months. If the patient is agitated and cannot relax enough to work or concentrate, sedating antidepressants like paroxetine (Paxil), trazodone (Desyrel), or amitriptyline (Elavil) could be used. If there are concerns related to a recent loss, such as the death of a loved one, referral to a grief counselor or other professional experienced in loss may be appropriate.

For patients who present with simple phobias, such as fear of cats, spiders, or elevators, a therapist competent in behavioral techniques might be the answer. Typically, various exposure techniques are preferred rather than medication for phobias.

TREATMENT REMINDERS AND CAUTIONS

For all patients with anxiety disorders, the therapist should advise them to eliminate or reduce the use of caffeine. In fact, patients may wish to evaluate their general diet and watch for excessive amounts of sugar or stimulants such as sodas, candy, and cigarettes.

For most anxiety disorders, the four "Bs" are used. These include: *benzodiazepines* such as diazepam (Valium), alprazolam (Xanax), lorazepam (Ativan), and clonazepam (Klonopin); *barbiturates* such as pentobarbital (Nembutal) and secobarbital (Seconal), which may potentiate GABA, but are very sedating and habit forming; *buspirone* (Buspar) for GAD; and *beta-blockers* for specific forms of social anxiety.

Side effects for anxiety medications vary according to the type used. Benzodiazepines are usually well tolerated and the side effects are minimal, but benzodiazepine intoxication includes slurred speech, severe sedation, dizziness, cognitive slowing, gait abnormalities, and an exaggerated sense of "high." Since some patients enjoy this feeling, therapists must watch for tolerance and abuse. Benzodiazepines should be given cautiously to seniors, because an excess may lead to falls and broken bones. Failure to assess the patient for a more serious depressive disorder or a psychotic disorder can result in a worsening of the condition when treated with benzodiazepines alone. The therapist should warn the patient that sudden withdrawal from benzodiazepines may cause an increase in anxiety and insomnia. Benzodiazepines should never be taken with alcohol, which will potentiate its effects. Tapering-off of the medication should be done gradually, under medical supervision, and only after the patient has discussed other options with the therapist and the prescribing professional.

The side effects for buspirone are usually mild and similar to those for antidepressants. They include drowsiness, dry mouth, nausea, headache, dizziness, and insomnia. As with the benzodiazepines, the patient must watch for dizziness, especially if operating heavy machinery.

Sleep aids should be used judiciously, that is, only when necessary and only for one to two weeks maximum if taken daily. In some cases patients may take sleep aids for long periods if they only use them for intermittent insomnia. Side effects are minimal, but include, of course, drowsiness, amnesia, dizziness, falling, lethargy, disorientation, cognitive slowing, and possible depression.

In conclusion, clinicians prescribing medication for anxiety disorders must make a quick and accurate assessment of the condition and have a sense of cooperation from their patients to assure proper dosing and compliance. Clinicians should obtain information about the duration and intensity of the condition, as well as history of substance abuse and previous treatment attempts.

CHAPTER EIGHT

TREATMENT OF PSYCHOTIC DISORDERS

In this chapter we will explore the various schizophrenia spectrum disorders, their prevalence, causes, and treatment. The role of both typical and atypical antipsychotics will be explored with advantages and disadvantages presented.

Topics to be addressed include the following:

- Schizophrenia spectrum disorders
- Causes of psychotic disorders
- Medication for psychotic behaviors
- Treatment protocol
- Other significant issues to consider

SCHIZOPHRENIA SPECTRUM DISORDERS

Schizophrenia and the other psychotic disorders affect more than 1 percent of the world's population and cost society a tremendous amount of resources (Sadock & Sadock, 2000). These authors also report that there are various schizophrenia spectrum disorders including schizoid personality disorder, schizotypal personality disorder, schizoaffective disorder, delusional disorder, and psychotic disorder NOS, which are reported to be less prevalent but still significant. Although hard data are scarce, Baethge (2002) reports the prevalence of schizoaffective disorder to be about 0.5 percent, one-half the prevalence of schizophrenia. Patients with schizophrenia need treatment in the earlier stages; this will help prevent relapse because of the higher morbidity and mortality associated with the earlier phases (Tandon and Jibson, 2003). In fact, Lambert, Conus, Lambert, and McGorry (2003) report that during the untreated phase and first-year treatment period, 10 to 15 percent of first-episode psychotic patients attempt suicide.

Schizophrenia

Schizophrenia is first and foremost a brain disease with numerous abnormalities in structure, function, and neurochemistry. With regards to brain structure, the most common finding is an enlargement of the lateral ventricles, followed by a decreased volume of gray and white matter. The medial temporal structures, including the hippocampus and amygdala, have been noted to be smaller in size when compared to normal brains. When looking at brain functioning, the clinician will note a relative decrease in cerebral blood flow and metabolism occuring in the frontal lobes.

Studies of the most common neurochemical abnormalities in patients with schizophrenia have focused on the dopamine hypothesis, which refers to the idea that *too much* dopamine is causing the psychotic symptoms. This is referred to as a *hyper-dopaminergic* hypothesis. As you may know, the conventional or typical antipsychotics (i.e., haloperidol or chlorpromazine), block postsynaptic dopamine D_2 receptors and reduce the symptoms of schizophrenia. The newer atypical antipsychotics (i.e., risperidone or olanzepine) have potent serotonergic $5-HT_2$ and dopaminergic D_2 antagonism. Other neurotransmitter systems that may be involved in schizophrenia include glutamate, acetylcholine, serotonin, norepinephrine, and other neuromodulators, such as substance P and neurotensin. These neuromodulators are localized with other neurochemicals and may influence their action. As noted in Chapter 2, their influence could facilitate, inhibit, or alter the patterns of firing.

As you may recall, schizophrenia and other schizophrenia spectrum disorders occur more commonly in families of patients with schizophrenia. Most researchers agree that monozygotic twins have a 40 to 50 percent concordance rate for schizophrenia, whereas dizygotic twins only have about a 10 percent concordance rate. This latter rate is consistent for the rate of occurrence of schizophrenia in other first-degree relatives.

In addition to the genetic theories for schizophrenia, immune and viral hypotheses also exist. In fact, some researchers believe that schizophrenia is more common in urban areas and in lower socioeconomic groups. This *social-drift* phenomenon refers to the fact that vulnerable patients have a tendency to lose their social and occupation status and *drift* toward pockets of poverty and inner city areas. Schizophrenia may have a north-to-south prevalence gradient in the Northern Hemisphere, whereas it may have a south-to-north gradient in the Southern Hemisphere. The illness may be endemic in a few areas, such as colder climates with patients born in winter months (Kendall and Adams, 1991).

When considering the viral hypotheses, reseachers suggest that a retrovirus could insert itself in the genome and alter the patient's genetic code; this altered code could be passed down through generations. Other mechanisms that might result in schizophrenia include: a viral infection in early life that creates a vulnerability toward the disease; a viral infection leading to secondary scar tissue formation; a virus triggering an autoimmune response; and so on. Some studies have reported that women exposed to the influenza virus during their second trimester are more likely to give birth to a child who is at increased risk for schizophrenia. The theory is that a viral infection may interfere with normal brain development during the active migration of neuronal cells (Sadock & Sadock, 2000).

Some researchers used to think that poor parenting could cause schizophrenia. In the 1950s, Harry Stack Sullivan (1953) focused on patients' disturbance that affected their capacity to relate to others, which is thought to reflect dysfunction in the mother-infant dyad. In the *stress-diathesis model*, various internal or external stressors can convert vulnerability for schizophrenia into symptoms.

Another concept worthy of mention is that of *expressed emotion* (EE). Several family factors including criticism, emotionally overinvolved attitudes and behaviors, and negative-affective style have been associated with precipitating the illness or aggravating its course. Schizophrenic patients living with families with high EE have a higher rate of relapse than those living in families with low EE. The chaotic and stressful family interactions might not be the cause of the dysfunction in schizophrenia, but rather the cause might be the complex collection of problems the patient brings to the family setting (Sadock & Sadock, 2000).

Symptoms in Schizophrenia

There are four different types of symptoms seen in schizophrenia and other psychotic illnesses: positive, negative, cognitive, and mood. Although there is a "classic" presentation, each patient is unique given the relative contribution from each of the four categories.

Positive Symptoms.   These symptoms involve a break from reality in the areas of perception, behavior, thought content, and thought processes. Hallucinations, delusions, loose associations, and grossly disorganized behavior are examples of positive symptoms. These symptoms may precipitate acute psychiatric hospitalizations.

Negative Symptoms.   Unlike positive symptoms, negative symptoms represent something that is deficient and may include apathy, blunted affect, amotivation, anhedonia, poverty of speech, poverty of thought content, asociality, ambivalence, poor hygiene, and so on. Although these symptoms cause the majority of functional disability associated with schizophrenia, negative symptoms rarely precipitate hospitalization.

Cognitive and Mood Symptoms.   The third type of symptoms to consider relate to *cognitive symptoms*. Schizophrenia is characterized by a broad impairment in cognition and neuropsychological functions, which correlates with functional impairment.

The fourth type of symptoms relates to *mood symptoms*. Some patients exhibit problems with depression, agitation, anxiety, insomnia, and mood lability.

When a patient is diagnosed with a psychotic illness, it is important to evaluate him or her properly for confounding factors such as substance abuse, medical illness, other psychiatric disorders, developmental disorders, and so on. The psychotic disorders include schizophrenia, schizophreniform disorder, schizoaffective disorder, delusional disorder, brief psychotic disorder, shared psychotic disorder, psychotic disorder due to a general medical condition, substance-induced psychotic disorder, and psychotic disorder NOS. When looking at schizophrenia more closely, there are five distinct subtypes defined by the predominant symptomatology: paranoid type, disorganized type, catatonic type, undifferentiated type, and residual type. Besides the psychotic disorders, other diagnoses may have secondary psychotic symptoms. For example, psychotic depression, postpartum depression, and bipolar disorder might possibly present with psychosis, depending on the level of severity. Later in this chapter, we will discuss treatment issues, which are similar among the various diagnoses.

CAUSES OF PSYCHOTIC DISORDERS

As with other psychiatric diagnoses, the etiology of a psychotic illness may be related to a physical rather than a functional disorder. The following is a list of common diseases that may cause or exacerbate psychosis:

Addison's disease (adrenal insufficiency)	Metabolic abnormalities
Brain tumors	Multiple sclerosis
CNS infections	Porphyria
Cushing's disease (hyperadrenalism)	Postoperative states
Delirium	Pregnancy/postpartum hormonal changes
Dementia (Alzheimer's, Parkinson's, etc.)	
Encephalitis (herpes, AIDS, neurosyphilis, etc.)	Stroke
	Systemic lupus erythematosus
Epilepsy	Traumatic brain injury
Huntington's disease	Uremia
Hyperthyroidism (thyrotoxicosis)	Vitamin deficiency (B_{12}, folate, or zinc)
Hypothyroidism (myxedema)	Wilson's Disease

In addition to the medical diagnoses, many medications and other substances have been associated with causing or exacerbating psychosis. The following is a list of these psychoactive substances:

Alcohol (intoxication or withdrawal)

Anticholinergic medications: benztropine, trihexyphenidyl, etc.

Antihistamines (diphenhydramine)

Antiparkinsonian medications: bromocriptine, amantadine, levodopa

Appetite suppressants (phentermine)

Barbiturates (intoxication or withdrawal)

Benzodiazepines (intoxication or withdrawal)

Beta-blockers: propranolol, metoprolol, atenolol

Corticosteroids and other hormones: prednisone, methylprednisolone androgens

Digoxin

Drugs of abuse: marijuana, amphetamines, PCP, psychedelics, cocaine, heroin/morphine, ephedra and other herbal stimulants

Environmental toxins: volatile hydrocarbons, organophosphates, and heavy metals

Narcotic medications: morphine, hydrocodone, etc.

Psychostimulant medications: dextroamphetamine, methylphenidate

Tricyclic antidepressants (TCAs)

After making a thorough assessment, establishing a differential diagnosis, and eliminating other causes for the psychosis, the therapist would plan an appropriate treatment protocol. While the mainstay of treatment for psychosis is pharmacotherapy, psychotherapy may still play an appropriate role. Although social skills training for the patient with schizophrenia may be helpful to improve communication skills, little evidence suggests that the behaviors generalize to improve social competence. However, broad-based training, such as the UCLA Social and Independent Living Skills, does enhance knowledge in specific areas studied (Huxley, Rendall, and Sederer, 2000). Researchers believe that the more specific training does generalize to improve social functioning. As expected, family therapy generally improves symptoms, decreases relapse, and improves social and occupational functioning. Individual, medication education sessions with the patient increase medication knowledge and treatment compliance. In addition, researchers overwhelmingly believe that a combination of family therapy and social skills training administered simultaneously works best.

MEDICATIONS FOR PSYCHOTIC BEHAVIORS

Although a wide range of treatment options is available for treating psychotic behaviors, expert-consensus guidelines recommend starting with the atypical antipsychotics. According to Kane, Leucht, Carpenter, and Docherty (2003), risperidone (Risperdal) is the treatment of choice for a first-episode psychotic patient with positive symptoms, negative symptoms, or a combination of both. Aripiprazole (Abilify), olanzepine (Zyprexa), ziprasidone (Geodon), and quetiapine (Seroquel) are additional choices but are secondary to the risperidone. You should note that these are all the newer atypical antipsychotic medications not the older typical (i.e., conventional) antipsychotics. Clozapine (Clozaril) was rated an excellent choice for second-line treatment after adequate trials of at least two of the atypical agents. See Table 8.1 for more information.

For multiepisode, psychotic patients, risperidone was again the treatment of choice regardless of predominating symptomatology. In addition to the other choices noted previously, Risperdal Consta, the only long-acting atypical antipsychotic, is considered an excellent second-line choice. Other less-desirable choices include a long-acting, intramuscular, conventional neuroleptic (such as Haldol or Prolixin Decanoate); an oral, high-potency neuroleptic, for example, haloperidol (Haldol); fluphenazine (Prolixin); trifluoperazine (Stelazine); or thiothixene (Navane). The oral, lower-potency, conventional, antipsychotic agents, such as chlorpromazine (Thorazine) and thioridazine (Mellaril), were less desirable to the experts when the literature was reviewed (Kane, Leucht et al., 2003) (see Table 8.2). Although acute treatment of agitation is not the focus here, two atypical antipsychotics that have an intramuscular formulation should be mentioned. Ziprasidone (Geodon IM) and

TABLE 8.1   Atypical Antipsychotic Medications

TRADE NAME	GENERIC NAME	TYPICAL DOSE (MG/DAY)	SEDATION	AUTONOMIC EFFECTS	EPS
Clozaril, Fazaclo	clozapine	400–600	***	***	None
Risperdal, Risperdal M-tab	risperidone	3–6	*	**	*
Risperdal Consta	risperidone	25–50 mg/ 2 weeks	*	*	*
Zyprexa, Zyprexa Zydis	olanzepine	10–20	**	**	*
Seroquel	quetiapine	300–600	***	***	*
Geodon	ziprasidone	80–160	*	**	*
Abilify	aripiprazole	10–30	*	*	*
Symbyax	olanzepine, fluoxetine	6/25–12/50	**	**	*

* Minimal, ** Moderate, ***Significant

olanzepine (Zyprexa IM) both have injectable forms of the medication used in emergency departments and acute psychiatric hospitals.

Atypical Antipsychotic Medications

The atypical antipsychotics have little or no EPS (dystonia, parkinsonism, akathisia, and tardive dyskinesia). Also, a broader spectrum of efficacy is thought to be associated with the newer agents. Benefits of the atypical antipsychotics agents versus the typical agents include:

- Minimal EPS
- Efficacy for positive symptoms (at least as effective as conventional agents)
- Improved efficacy for negative symptoms
- Improved cognition
- Improved mood

Although the atypical agents have similar efficacy, the side-effect profiles have been found to be quite different. Tandon and Jibson (2003) report risperidone (Risperdal) shows a clear dose-related increase in EPS and prolactin level, especially above 6 mg daily. Prolactin is a hormone secreted by the pituitary gland that increases

TABLE 8.2 Typical or Conventional Antipsychotic Medications

TRADE NAME	GENERIC NAME	TYPICAL DOSE (MG/DAY)	SEDATION	AUTONOMIC EFFECTS	EPS
Thorazine	chlorpromazine	200–600	***	***	**
Mellaril	thioridazine	200–600	***	***	**
Serentil	mesoridazine	50–400	***	***	*
Loxitane	loxapine	20–100	**	*	**
Trilafon	perphenazine	8–64	**	*	**
Moban	molindone	20–100	**	*	**
Navane	thiothixene	5–30	*	*	***
Stelazine	trifluoperazine	5–30	*	*	***
Prolixin	fluphenazine	2–20	*	*	***
Prolixin Decanoate	fluphenazine decanoate	25–50 mg/ 2 wks	*	*	**
Haldol	haloperidol	2–20	*	*	***
Haldol Decanoate	haloperidol decanoate	100–300 mg/ month	*	*	**
Orap	pimozide	1–10	*	*	***

*Minimal, **Moderate, ***Significant

when dopamine is blocked or suppressed. Increased prolactin concentrations may lead to breast enlargement, galactorrhea (production of breast milk), irregular menses, and so on. Patients who receive increasing doses of olanzepine (Zyprexa) will likely exhibit akathisia, parkinsonism, modest prolactin elevation, and weight gain. The use of ziprasidone (Geodon) shows a trend toward an increasing use of anticholinergic medication at higher doses (Daniel, Zimbroff, Potkin, Reeves, Harrigan, & Lakshminarayan, 1999). Quetiapine (Seroquel) tends to be similar to a placebo when considering weight, prolactin levels, and EPS. Clozapine (Clozaril) results in the most weight gain and sedation of all the agents. Keep in mind that clozapine requires weekly blood monitoring and more intense supervision (see Chapter 6).

Typical Antipsychotic Medications

The typical neuroleptics have similar efficacy with respect to positive symptoms, but they may worsen negative symptoms because of their side-effect profiles. Extrapyramidal symptoms have a tremendous negative impact on treatment. *Acute dystonic reactions* are uncomfortable, frightening, and lead to poor compliance. Bradykinesia, cogwheel rigidity, and stiffness, which are *parkinsonism* side effects, contribute to the negative symptoms of the illness (i.e., reducing facial expression, affective responses, gestures, and vocal intonation) from which the patient is already struggling. *Akathisia* is a common subacute side effect related to these medications and may be experienced as restlessness, anxiety, agitation, or insomnia. *Tardive dyskinesia* is the major chronic extrapyramidal symptom that should be avoided if at all possible. The typical agents also have a negative impact on cognition, which further impairs the patient's ability to think and function independently. EPS is commonly treated with antiparkinsonian or anticholinergic medications that may also interfere with cognition (see Table 8.3). All of these side effects contribute to discontinuing therapy and long-term compliance issues.

Adverse Effects of Typical Antipsychotics

Adverse drug reactions may be seen with any prescribed or over-the-counter medication. As noted in Table 8.2, typical antipsychotics vary with their ability to cause side effects including sedation, autonomic effects, and extrapyramidal symptoms (EPS). Autonomic side effects refer to the adverse effect of medications on the autonomic nervous system and include dizziness, hypotension, and flushing.

The typical or conventional antipsychotics are known for their EPS effects, which include acute dystonia, parkinsonism, akathisia, and tardive dyskinesia. An acute dystonic reaction may occur immediately following a dose of medication and involves intermittent and/or sustained spasms of the muscles of the trunk, head, and neck. Dystonias usually occur within hours to days of the medication and typically are very frightening for the patient.

Parkinsonism, the second form of EPS, may include rigidity, bradykinesia, shuffling gait, and tremor. Patients who take dopamine receptor blockers may look like they have idiopathic Parkinson's disease. This side effect usually occurs within days to weeks of starting the antipsychotic medications.

TABLE 8.3   Antiparkinsonian and Anticholinergic Medications

TRADE NAME	GENERIC NAME	TYPICAL DOSE (MG/DAY)	CHEMICAL CLASS
Benadryl	diphenhydramine	25–50	antihistamine
Symmetrel	amantadine	100–300	dopamine agonist
Inderal, Inderal LA	propranolol	40–80	beta-blocker
Valium	diazepam	5–10	benzodiazepine
Ativan	lorazepam	1–3	benzodiazepine
Klonopin	clonazepam	1–3	benzodiazepine
Cogentin	benztropine	2–6	anticholinergic
Artane	trihexyphenidyl	5–15	anticholinergic

The most common extrapyramidal side effect is called akathisia, which translates to inability to sit still. Akathisia usually presents itself clinically as feelings of inner restlessness, inability to keep the legs still, constant shifting of weight from one foot to the other, walking in place, frequent shifting of body positions in a chair, and so on. Like parkinsonism side effects, akathisia typically occurs after days to weeks of treatment. Acute dystonia, parkinsonism, and akathisia occur early in treatment with the typical antipsychotics and remit soon after the drug is discontinued.

The last type of EPS is tardive dyskinesia (TD). It is an involuntary movement disorder that may occur after the patient has been on the medication for months to years. Patients with TD may have abnormal movements including lip smacking, sucking or puckering, facial grimacing, blinking, tremors, trunk movements, and so on. The risk for developing tardive dyskinesia is approximately 10 to 20 percent of patients who are treated with dopamine receptor antagonists for more than a year. Certain populations such as elderly females and patients with mood disorders are at greater risk.

TREATMENT PROTOCOL

The following general steps simplify the treatment information, which may be a bit overwhelming and confusing.

Step 1. Most prescribing professionals will start with risperidone (Risperdal) or similar atypical agent for the patient's psychotic illness.

Step 2. If the patient is unable to tolerate risperidone because of side effects or does not respond, the next logical choices would be olanzepine (Zyprexa), quetiapine (Seroquel), ziprasidone (Geodon), or aripiprazole (Abilify). Preferably, the clinician should try two or more of the atypical agents before moving on to the next steps.

Step 3. This step varies and depends on the art of medicine. Some clinicians would recommend a trial of clozapine (Clozaril), while others would use a typical antipsychotic medication like haloperidol (Haldol) or thiothixene (Navane).

Step 4. Another option the clinician could try is to add a third agent in the atypical antipsychotic class. Remember that the long-acting typical antipsychotics (e.g., Haldol Decanoate or Prolixin Decanoate) are also available for patients who have compliance issues.

OTHER SIGNIFICANT ISSUES TO CONSIDER

In addition to choosing the most appropriate medication, other issues must be considered. An *adequate dose* of the antipsychotic, which is approximately the dose recommended in the package labeling, must be prescribed. For example, the optimal dose of risperidone would be in the range of 4–6 mg daily, whereas the dose for olanzepine would be 15–30 mg daily. Each drug has a different dose because of different potencies, but they are all equally efficacious at therapeutic doses. For chronic patients, the doses of the medications may be higher than for first-episode patients.

Information on *therapeutic drug monitoring* with the antipsychotics is limited. Clozapine is the only agent where researchers have considered the plasma level most clinically useful. Some experts believe that plasma levels of other neuroleptics can be useful to aid in dosage adjustment, especially when there is an inadequate response or problematic side effects.

Research indicates that a relationship exists between certain patient characteristics and necessary dose adjustments. First, smoking can reduce the plasma levels of some antipsychotics drugs (Van Der Weide, Steijns, & Van Weelden, 2003). A body of mounting evidence suggests that the effects of genetic polymorphisms involve cytochrome P450 liver enzymes and the metabolism of psychotropic drugs. Ethnicity, sex, age, and other medical conditions may be factors in determining the best dose for the patient. For example, geriatric patients and Asian patients who tend to be more sensitive to antipsychotic medications require lower dosages because of their slower metabolic processes in the liver.

Since the patient's response to these medications is delayed, an *adequate treatment trial* is important. Expert consensus guidelines recommend waiting a minimum of three weeks and a maximum of six weeks before making a major change in the treatment regimen (Kane et al., 2003). Some prescribers wait longer than six weeks if the patient is showing a partial response, especially during the second or subsequent trials.

When switching from one atypical agent to another, most prescribers recommend cross-titration as opposed to overlap and taper. *Cross-titration* refers to gradually tapering down the dose of the first agent while gradually increasing the dose of the second antipsychotic. In contrast, *overlap* and *taper* refer to continuing the same dose of the first drug while gradually increasing the second drug to a therapeutic level and then tapering the first.

As with the antidepressants, the antipsychotic medications may also be augmented if the patient has a partial response. A combination of an atypical antipsychotic and a mood stabilizer has been used clinically despite the lack of empirical evidence in the literature. Some prescribers use combinations of two atypical antipsychotics agents or one atypical agent and one conventional antipsychotic. Again, there is lack of data to support these practices. The various combinations of medications usually lead to an increased number of side effects as well as excessive cost. Symbyax is an example of a combination drug that consists of fluoxetine (Prozac) and olanzepine (Zyprexa) in varying doses. This may be useful in patients with schizophrenia and depression or the depressive phase of bipolar disorder.

Clozapine (Clozaril) is indicated for treatment-refractory schizophrenia. Most clinicians define *treatment refractory* as failing to respond to one or more conventional antipsychotics and two atypical antipsychotics. In addition, approximately 30 to 50 percent of treatment-refractory patients will respond to clozapine. In some instances, ECT may be considered after other options have been exhausted. Remember that the primary goals of treatment are rapid and complete control of acute psychotic symptoms, avoidance of functional deterioration, and prevention of relapse.

CHAPTER NINE

TREATMENT OF
ADHD AND DISORDERS
OF ATTENTION

This chapter explores the nature and causes of ADHD and other disorders of attention. Special consideration is given to diagnosis and matching the right behavioral and pharmacological treatment to the needs of patients and their families.

Topics to be addressed include the following:

- Etiology of ADHD
- Diagnostic assessment of attention disorders
- Psychological and pharmacological treatment

Attention deficit disorders are the most common disorders presenting in childhood. Researchers estimate that approximately 3 to 7 percent of all school-age children have attention deficit disorders (Kratochvil, Vaughan, Harrington & Burke, 2003; Spencer, Biederman, Wilens & Faraone, 2002). Further, they estimate that as many as 70 percent of these youth will demonstrate ADD or ADHD symptoms into their adult years (Aviram, Rhum & Levin, 2001; McCann & Roy-Byrne, 2000). While the symptoms for adults with these disorders are almost identical to the symptoms seen in children, adults tend to display less hyperactivity and more internalized restlessness.

Treatment of ADHD can be complicated, because many children who meet diagnostic criteria for the disorder may also have comorbid oppositional and conduct disorders (Wilson & Levin, 2001). Wilson and Levin also estimated that approximately 50 percent of youth treated for substance abuse meet diagnostic criteria for ADHD. Some clinicians are concerned that treating ADHD with stimulants may increase the risk for substance abuse including possibly abusing the stimulant, but research suggests that treating ADHD early may in fact reduce this risk (Aviram et al. 2001; Wilson & Levin, 2001). Animal studies have indicated that stimulants such as methylphenidate are far less likely to be abused than other stimulants such as cocaine (Kollins, 2003). Further, Kollins found that an ADHD patient is less likely to abuse methylphenidate and other therapeutic stimulants than those without the diagnosis

ETIOLOGY OF ADHD

Molecular genetics and neuroimaging studies confirm that disorders of attention like ADHD are heterogeneous, neurobiological disorders, mainly of dopaminergic and noradrenergic pathways (Adler & Chua, 2002). These researchers further found as much as a 50 percent concordance rate with other first-degree relatives. Subsequent studies have further demonstrated frontal lobe dysfunction in the pathophysiology of ADHD and a dysregulation of the neurotransmitters dopamine and norepinephrine in the frontal lobes, the basil ganglia, the amygdala, and possibly the reticular formation (Zimmerman, 2003). Functional MRI scans have consistently shown irregular neurotransmitter activity in the frontal striatal networks and in the anterior cingulate gyrus (Weiss & Murry, 2003). These areas of the brain also act like filters, assisting the patient in screening out irrelevant information from important information. Drugs used in the treatment of attention disorders *stimulate* these brain centers, allowing them to work faster and more efficiently. This stimulation assists the patient with both attention and retention of information.

DIAGNOSTIC ASSESSMENT OF ATTENTION DISORDERS

While attention-disorder symptoms for adults and children are essentially similar, adults may exhibit less hyperactivity and more reports of restlessness and agitation. As stated in the DSM-IV diagnostic criteria, considering a childhood history of ADD or ADHD is necessary for the adult diagnosis. A strong family history is usually found. Another important item to remember is the DSM-IV criterion that requires the patient to demonstrate symptoms and behaviors in more than one setting. Various testing and evaluation instruments can assist in making the diagnosis. Many professionals use the Conner's Rating Scales-Revised, the Conner's Adult ADHD Rating Scales, The Attention Deficit/Hyperactivity Disorder Test, or the ADHD Problem Checklist. Once again, to determine if the patient truly has the disorder, the clinician should review all of the DSM criteria and rule out another axis I or II condition or learning disability and perhaps the existence of a physical condition such as thyroid abnormalities that could contribute to these symptoms.

PSYCHOLOGICAL AND PHARMACOLOGICAL TREATMENT

Only a few controlled studies have considered the efficacy of psychological treatments for ADHD. Most available studies have emphasized the need for social-skills training, time-management techniques, vocational and career appraisal, and life coaching in addition to addressing poor self-esteem and other stereotypes experienced by these patients (Bemporad, 2001; Weiss & Murray, 2003). These authors and others stress the need for daily coping strategies, including meal planning, conflict resolution, and parenting skills. Good patient education is also necessary to help patients and their families understand the condition and to formulate realistic expectations (Barkley, 2002).

The best treatment approach for attention disorders involves both a psychological and pharmacological approach. The use of stimulants and other antidepressants that potentiate levels of dopamine and norepinephrine show the greatest promise. Table 9.1 lists the psychostimulants used in the treatment of ADHD. These are the same stimulants mentioned in Chapter 5 for augmentation of antidepressants. These medications tend to be dose dependent, that is, higher doses typically correspond to better response rates. Typical side effects include hypertension, insomnia, headaches, weight loss, and growth retardation in children. Insomnia is usually controlled by using stimulants with shorter half-lives that wear off before bedtime.

As clinicians know, the potential for abuse with stimulants is high, and they may need to determine the risk of using these substances with patients who have a history of abuse. Also, patients who are taking MAOIs; lithium; neuroleptics such as haloperidol (Haldol) and chlorpromazine (Thorazine); certain antidepressants such as amitriptyline (Elavil), nortriptyline (Pamelor), and imipramine (Tofranil); and certain analgesics should refrain from using stimulants unless they are monitored closely.

TABLE 9.1   Psychostimulant Medications

TRADE NAME	GENERIC NAME	CHILD/ADULT TYPICAL DOSE (MG/DAY)	LEVEL OF INSOMNIA
Adderall,	amphetamine/mixed	5–30/5–60	**
Adderall-XR	salts		***
Cylert	pemoline	37.5–112.5	**
Dexedrine	dextroamphetamine	5–10/5–60	*
Dextrostat			
Dexedrine Spansules			**
Desoxyn	methamphetamine	5–25/5–30	*
Ritalin[1]	methylphenidate	10–30/10–40	*
Ritalin-SR			**
Methylin-ER			**
Metadate-ER[2]			**
Concerta[3]		18–54	***
Focalin[1]	dexmethylphenidate	5–30/5–40	*

[1]Effective for 2–6 hours

[2]Effective for 6–8 hours

[3]Once per day dosing

* Mild ** Moderate *** Significant

If the patient is a child who needs to be able to focus during school, after school, and for evening homework, the clinician should consider the longer-acting stimulants such as Adderall XR (a brand of amphetamine salts) and Concerta (a brand of methylphenidate). If the child has problems with sleeping, the clinician should consider stimulants with shorter half-lives such as standard dextroamphetamine (Dexedrine) or methylphenidate (Ritalin). The longer-acting stimulants such as Metadate ER and Ritalin SR (i.e., types of methylphenidate) have a polymer, multiparticulate bead system that allows for breakdown and delivery over several hours. Concerta is a bit more ambitious. It has an outer capsule that delivers an immediate dose and an inner core that is released over twelve hours by gastrointestinal pressure through a laser-drilled hole in the membrane. Once empty, the capsule is passed in the stool.

Any patient with ADHD should see a physician for a complete physical. Patients with glaucoma, hypertension, and tic disorders should be evaluated and counseled by their primary care physician before starting stimulants.

In addition to the psychostimulants, antidepressants and alpha-adrenergic agonists are used in the treatment of ADHD (see Table 9.2). As mentioned in Chapter 5, antidepressants need to be prescribed cautiously for children and adolescents because of the FDA warning about an increase in suicide thinking and behaviors. For more complete information on medication side effects, see Chapter 5 or the Appendix.

Many experts who treat patients with ADHD have found that a combination of psychotherapy, stimulants, and antidepressants offer a complete and direct treatment approach to the condition. While stimulants work for most patients, in some cases antidepressants offer symptom relief. Atomoxetine (Strattera) or antidepressants with stimulating qualities often are prescribed alone for the condition. Bupropion (Wellbutrin) is most often the antidepressant of choice, because it does not interfere with

TABLE 9.2   Typical Antidepressants and Alpha-Adrenergic Agonists Used in the Treatment of ADHD

TRADE NAME	GENERIC NAME	TYPICAL DOSE (MG/DAY)
Effexor, Effexor XR	venlafaxine	50–300/75–300
Norpramin	desipramine	150–300
Pamelor	nortriptyline	75–125
Wellbutrin, Wellbutrin SR, Wellbutrin XL	bupropion	75–450/100–400/150–450
Strattera	atomoxetine	40–100
Catapres	clonidine	0.2–0.9
Tenex	guanfacine	1–9

most stimulants and offers enriched levels of dopamine and norepinephrine. Medications are typically given with titration of doses upward until complete symptomatic relief is noticed. It is not uncommon for parents to request drug holidays for children in the nonschool, summer months. This practice often helps allow growing periods for the child since many stimulants can stunt growth.

Many parents today are concerned about placing their child on drugs, especially stimulants. They will often cite newspaper articles and pieces from popular magazines suggesting that behavioral therapy alone is sufficient. Some parents believe that diet alone will improve their child's symptoms. While sugary snacks certainly do not help children with ADHD, the connection between sweets and behavior is not conclusive. In most cases, children and adults with moderate-to-severe cases of ADHD do not respond adequately to dietary changes, behavioral interventions, and environmental changes alone. The clinician should educate the parents and the patient about the benefits of medications. The proof will be noticed in the child's behavior and academic performance, and nothing else, aside from counseling, is better for raising self-esteem and assuring a healthy sense of independence.

CHAPTER TEN

TREATMENT OF COGNITIVE DISORDERS

This chapter presents a discussion of the various forms and causes of dementia, and how best to treat them and reduce the negative aspects caused by these conditions. The advantages and disadvantages of various medications for cognitive decline will be explored and discussed.

Topics to be addressed include the following

- Forms of dementia
- Alzheimer's disease
- Medical and behavioral evaluation
- Medications for cognitive disorders
- Other approaches to cognitive enhancement
- Other significant issues to consider

The cognitive disorders consist of delirium and dementia, although this chapter will focus mainly on dementia. Delirium is an acute confusional state that is basically a medical emergency; the patient needs acute medical treatment to find the etiology of the confusion and treat it accordingly. For the most part, delirium would not be part of a patient's clinical presentation to your treatment settings. On the other hand, dementia is becoming more of an issue as our population ages. Alzheimer's disease (AD), the most common type of dementia, affects more than 15 million people worldwide; the United States has about 4 million people with the disease (Grossberg, 2003). In fact, Brookmeyer, Gray, and Kawas (1998) have suggested the prevalence of AD in the United States would rise to approximately 9.3 million over the next fifty years. Grossberg further reports this would translate to about 1 in 45 Americans with AD.

FORMS OF DEMENTIA

Dementia has many different forms that include memory disturbance as their central feature. The three most common forms are: Alzheimer's disease, dementia with Lewy bodies, and vascular dementia.

Alzheimer's disease accounts for approximately 60 percent of all irreversible dementias. It will be discussed as the prototype for our purposes although other less-common diagnoses may be treated in a similar fashion. In addition to the memory problems, Alzheimer's disease is characterized by either aphasia, apraxia, and/or agnosia. Dementia with Lewy bodies (DLB) is the second most common type of dementia accounting for about 20 to 25 percent; it is characterized by memory dysfunction with visual hallucinations, parkinsonism, and/or fluctuating alertness levels. Of note, dementia with Lewy bodies and another cause of dementia, Parkinson's disease, probably have similar neuropathology. Vascular dementia is the third most common type but accounts for less than 20 percent overall. Classically, vascular dementia was thought to be the second most common type ahead of DLB and was previously known as multiinfarct dementia (MID). The less-common forms of dementia include the following: frontotemporal dementia (i.e., Pick's disease), corticobasal degeneration, progressive supranuclear palsy, Creutzfeldt-Jakob disease, neurosyphilis, normal-pressure hydrocephalus, and HIV-associated dementia (Boeve, Silber, & Ferman, 2002).

Overall these disorders are a significant public health concern because of their economic burden. Grossberg (2003) reports the estimated annual cost of AD in the United States to be in the range of $67 billion. Of the total costs, direct patient care accounts for 31 percent, lost productivity due to illness or premature mortality accounts for 20 percent, and unpaid caregiver cost is the remaining 49 percent. As the number of patients and the cost to society increases, we will all be facing this issue at some point, either professionally or personally.

ALZHEIMER'S DISEASE

Alzheimer's disease is characterized by gradual onset and marked by progressive decline in cognition; motor function declines in the later stages. Research indicates that several neurotransmission pathways may be involved including *cholinergic, glutamatergic, serotonergic, and dopaminergic.* At this point in time, loss of cholinergic neurons appears to be the most important abnormality. In the mid 1970s, researchers discovered a deficit in brain presynaptic cholinergic systems in postmortem brain tissue in patients with AD (Davies & Maloney, 1976). This discovery has led to a major finding: Acetylcholinesterase inhibitors, which increase intrasynaptic acetylcholine levels, produce moderate symptomatic improvement in AD.

Inflammatory processes may also play a role in the disease progression. Senile plaques consisting of beta-amyloid are the most widely studied neuropathologic change in AD. These plaques do not affect the whole nervous system uniformly, but only certain vulnerable cortical and subcortical areas; the sensory and motor regions of the brain tend to remain unaffected. Chronic neuroinflammation may be responsible for the degeneration of cholinergic neurons via a chain of inflammatory processes initiated by beta-amyloid.

Sometimes a faulty gene may cause the problem, which is the familial form of AD. On the other hand, the more common form of the disease is known as sporadic AD. The genes that contribute to AD appear in all cells but their expression varies in different areas of the brain and in different individuals. Obviously, the neuroanatomy and neurochemistry is very complex and beyond the scope of this chapter. We just wanted to give you some hint of these issues.

MEDICAL AND BEHAVIORAL EVALUATION OF COGNITIVE DISORDERS

As part of the medical evaluation of the cognitive disorders, an inventory of current prescribed and other-the-counter medications needs to be reviewed and analyzed as potential causes. Behavioral toxicity associated with pharmacotherapy is the most common etiology of reversible delirium. Appropriate laboratory evaluation including serum electrolytes, blood urea nitrogen (BUN) levels, serum B_{12} level, and thyroid-function tests should be done. Vitamin B_{12} deficiency and hypothyroidism may present as reversible causes of a cognitive disorder if detected in the earlier stages. A diagnostic neuroimaging procedure (CT or MRI of the brain) is commonly used to rule out tumors, subdural hematomas, and normal-pressure hydrocephalus. The clinician should obtain a past psychiatric history from the patient or family, because patients with major mental illness can also develop dementia in later life (e.g., schizophrenia complicated by AD).

While the medical aspects of cognitive disorders are important, the clinician also needs to look at behavioral factors that precipitate or contribute to some of the dysfunction. Patients with dementia who have poor short-term memory and disorientation may appear quite compensated as long as they remain in a familiar environment that does not require new learning. Furthermore, when these patients are moved to a hospital, nursing home, or other unfamiliar setting, they may become disoriented and disorganized, leading to physical aggression and acting out. Once the patient adapts to the new environment, behavioral problems may resolve spontaneously over a month or so. If aphasia is part of the dementia, patients will have difficulty expressing themselves. This difficulty may present as grabbing or aggressive behaviors when a patient is in pain or needs to go to the restroom. Patients who are apraxic may be unable to carry out their routine activities of daily living, which leads to agitation and/or low-frustration tolerance. In addition, family and staff visits are not always welcomed by the patient. If any particular behavior patterns arise, hospital or nursing home staff may need to observe interactions and determine the triggers of these behavior problems (Goldberg, 2002).

MEDICATIONS FOR COGNITIVE DISORDERS

Only a few approved medications are available for treatment of Alzheimer's disease (see Table 10.1). These drugs improve cognitive function only modestly; however, they are best conceptualized as drugs that "stabilize" cognition, activities of daily living, and behavioral function. Basically, the cholinesterase inhibitors slow the clinical

TABLE 10.1 Medications for Cognitive Disorders

TRADE NAME	GENERIC NAME	TYPICAL DOSE (MG/DAY)	CHEMICAL CLASS
Cognex	tacrine	40–160	cholinesterase inhibitor
Aricept	donepezil	5–10	cholinesterase inhibitor
Exelon	rivastigmine	6–12	cholinesterase inhibitor
Reminyl	galantamine	16–24	cholinesterase inhibitor
Namenda	memantine	10–20	NMDA receptor antagonists

deterioration in AD, but they do not cure it. In the early 1990s, tacrine (Cognex) was the first cholinesterase inhibitor demonstrated to be effective in the treatment of AD. Unfortunately, liver toxicity has significantly limited its use in treatment.

Second-generation cholinesterase inhibitors, such as donepezil (Aricept), have been shown to be as effective as tacrine without the hepatic toxicity. Donepezil has shown positive effects on cognition and overall functioning in AD patients with mild-to-moderate disease (Rogers & Friedhoff, 1996). This medication is easy to use, because it is given once daily and has only two therapeutic doses, 5 mg or 10 mg. As with all the cholinesterase inhibitors, the most common side effects are gastrointestinal symptoms including nausea, vomiting, and diarrhea. Donepezil also appears to extend its benefit into more advanced stages of AD than initially thought. Feldman, Gauthier, Hector and colleagues (2001) showed significant benefit in moderate to severe AD with continued good tolerability as far as side effects.

Rivastigmine (Exelon) is another medication used in treatment of AD. In addition to inhibiting acetylcholinesterase, rivastigmine inhibits butyrylcholinesterase. The clinical meaningfulness of this latter effect remains to be determined, but butyryl-cholinesterase appears to regulate brain acetylcholine levels in animal studies (Blazer, Steffens, & Busse, 2004). Gastrointestinal effects of rivastigimine occur in up to 40 percent of patients, which is more common than with donepezil. Some evidence suggests that rivastigmine may be effective with behavioral problems that are particularly prominent in dementia with Lewy bodies.

The final cholinesterase inhibitor is galantamine (Reminyl), which also modulates the nicotinic acetylcholine receptor responsiveness at an allosteric binding site (Blazer et al. 2004). Because a prominent nicotinic cholinergic deficit exists in AD, this additional benefit may be clinically useful. The dosage titration with galantamine is more cumbersome with the maximum dose being 24 mg/d. The side-effect profile looks similar to donepezil if galantamine is slowly increased to a therapeutic dose.

Another class of medications being used is N-methyl-D-aspartate (NMDA) receptor antagonists. According to the glutamate excitotoxicity hypothesis, beta-amyloid indirectly stimulates the production of excessive glutamate; glutamate in turn over-stimulates the NMDA receptors. This process results in neuronal death because of the chronic excitation. To reduce the negative effect of glutamate, experts theorize that intervening as early as possible in the process of AD would help the patient most. Glutamate is thought to play a more prominent role in the early stages of AD rather than the late stages. A medication called memantine (Namenda) was approved in late 2003 for use in AD. The most common side effects of memantine include agitation, urinary incontinence, urinary tract infection, and insomnia. Tariot, Farlow, Grossberg, and colleagues (2004) have reported that memantine, when used in combination with cholinesterase inhibitors, may be useful in patients with more moderate to severe AD.

OTHER APPROACHES TO COGNITIVE ENHANCEMENT

Vitamin E and other antioxidants have been used to slow the progression of aging and dementia (Sano, Ernesto, et. al., 1997). Vitamin E may slow the deterioration associated with AD, but not necessarily in the cognitive domain. Some studies found that antioxidants were more effective than placebo in delaying deterioration to functional endpoints such as nursing home placement or substantial loss of daily-living activities. The dose of Vitamin E recommended in the studies was 1,000 IU given twice daily.

Another medication to consider is selegiline (Eldepryl), which is a selective inhibitor of monoamine oxidase. This medication is used most commonly in Parkinson's disease but may also be used for depression given that it is an MAOI. The doses of selegiline used in the studies were 10–40 mg daily. As with Vitamin E, treatment with selegiline slows functional deterioration but has little effect on cognitive decline.

Extracts of the leaf of the ginkgo biloba tree have been used in traditional Chinese medications and may have antioxidant, anti-inflammatory, and stimulant properties. A standardized extract of ginkgo biloba has been studied; the results show a small but statistically significant effect on cognitive functioning (Le Bars, Katz, et. al, 1997). The improvement was approximately one-half of the effect seen with the cholinesterase inhibitors. Currently, ginko biloba is being studied further to evaluate its effectiveness and usefulness.

Studies in postmenopausal women suggest that estrogen replacement therapy decreases the risk of AD for this population. Evidence is still conflicting as to whether conjugated estrogens or more naturally occurring forms are neuroprotective. Keep in mind that treatment with estrogens may also increase the risk of heart disease and breast cancer (Warren, 2004).

Research suggests that nonsteroidal anti-inflammatory drugs (NSAIDS) might decrease the risk of AD in some patients. By decreasing the inflammation caused by the plaques containing beta-amyloid, the neurons have less damage and cell death. Unfortunately, the potent, anti-inflammatory steroid prednisone failed to show any positive effect on cognition or disease progression (Aisen 2002). Trials using naproxen (Naprosyn) and rofecoxib (Vioxx) have also been negative. Rofecoxib has been withdrawn from worldwide markets because of the increase risk of heart attack and stroke. Some clinicians have suggested that certain types of NSAIDS and aspirin may decrease beta-amyloid production, while other types do not. At this point in time, the use of NSAIDS and aspirin does not seem promising in the treatment of AD; however, they may be helpful in prevention.

Agents that lower cholesterol may be useful in preventing AD. Lipid-lowering agents, such as various statin drugs, are associated with a decrease in central nervous system amyloid deposition in animal models (Sano, 2003). Atorvastatin (Lipitor), simvastatin (Zocor), and pravastatin (Pravachol) are common examples of statins. Clinical trials are currently underway to evaluate their usefulness in the treatment of AD.

OTHER SIGNIFICANT ISSUES TO CONSIDER

Behavioral complications of dementia include physical agitation, verbal aggression, physical aggression, depression, and psychosis. An organized way to approach patients with behavioral problems is to define some *target symptoms*, which will dictate the treatment protocol. For example, an atypical antipsychotic agent would be considered as a starting point for an AD patient presenting with agitation, aggression, or psychotic symptoms. Risperidone (Risperdal) has been effective in this situation with dosages up to 2 mg with minimal side effects. However, the use of atypical antipsychotic medications in the elderly has been associated with an increase in cerebrovascular events (stroke and transient ischemic attacks) and even death. Typical antipsychotic medications, such as haloperidol (Haldol) or chlorpromazine (Thorazine), should be avoided if possible, because they present a high risk of tardive dyskinesia (TD) in the elderly (see Chapter 8 for more information on TD). Another option for a patient with agitation would be the mood stabilizers. Carbamazepine (Tegretol) and valproate (Depakote) have both been used in low-to-moderate doses with overall decrease in agitation. If an AD patient primarily has depressive and anxiety symptoms, an SSRI would be an excellent choice. The information regarding these medications discussed in previous chapters will be applicable here. Of note, caution should be used in medicating elderly patients given the high prevalence of polypharmacy and multiple medical diagnoses.

Except for Alzheimer's disease the, data is sparse on the treatment of other dementia syndromes. Vascular dementia, for example, occurs rarely in isolation. More commonly, a combination of two neuropathological processes may occur together, which is referred to as a *mixed dementia*. These types of dementias may respond to the treatment options suggested for Alzheimer's disease alone.

CHAPTER ELEVEN

TREATMENT OF SLEEP DISORDERS

This chapter thoroughly explores sleep disturbances, primary sleep disorders and parasomnias. Various treatment issues and options will be presented and discussed.

Topics to be addressed include the following:

- Stages of sleep
- Sleep disorders and conditions
- Behavioral techniques for treating sleep disorders
- Pharmacology for sleep disorders
- Holistic treatments

Sleep disturbances are a frequently cited problem by mental health patients. While many of these patients also have comorbid physical conditions that interfere with the quality of their sleep, many have other Axis I and/or Axis II conditions that cause sleep disturbances secondary to mental health conditions. Some patients experience sleep disturbances related to substance use or abuse. Research has established that those with sleep disorders are at increased risk for developing hypertension and suffering cardiovascular morbidity and mortality (Richert & Baran, 2003). The most common sleep complaints made by mental health patients involve initial insomnia (difficulty falling asleep) or intermittent awakening throughout the night (middle insomnia). Some patients may fall asleep normally but awaken very early in the morning with difficulty falling back to sleep (terminal insomnia). A national survey of more than 1000 adults studied by researchers found that 43 percent reported middle-of-the-night awakening, of which 26 percent could not return to sleep and 34 percent complained of daytime fatigue. A similar study found that as many as 56 percent had difficulty with initial insomnia, and 67 percent experienced intermittent awakening (Scharf, 2001).

STAGES OF SLEEP

There are five distinct stages of sleep. Stages 1 and 2, the theta stages, are rather light stages of sleep. If patients' names are called out during these stages they would probably awaken without feeling groggy. People spend about 50 percent of sleep time in stages 1 and 2.

Stages 3 and 4 are called the delta stages of sleep, which are characterized by slow-wave patterns and very deep, restorative sleep. Here, shaking the patient is necessary to awaken him or her, and the patient would be groggy. People spend about 20 percent of their sleep time in these stages.

Stage 5 is the rapid-eye-movement or REM stage. It occupies about 25 percent of the night and is characterized by both theta- and beta-type activity that resembles the wave patterns seen while awake. Most dreams occur during this stage. If patients are sleep deprived, they will demonstrate additional time spent in stages 3, 4, and REM during their next sleep period, which is called the *rebound phenomenon* (Carlson, 2004). Serotonin is necessary to maintain adequate sleep, especially in stages 1–4. Norepinephrine is necessary for REM sleep, so not surprisingly, depressed patients with lower levels of serotonin and norepinephrine experience problems with the quality of their sleep.

When discussing sleep concerns with a patient, the clinician needs to determine if the patient has a primary sleep disturbance, that is, a sleep disorder that is not caused by a medical, psychiatric, or substance-abuse related issue. In such cases, the clinician must collect adequate history information to assure that no other complicating conditions or factors exist. The clinician should inquire about such issues as daytime sleepiness, memory/concentration concerns, depression, an increase in accidents, and impaired job functioning. Referral to a neurologist or sleep specialist may be in order to determine the cause.

SLEEP DISORDERS AND CONDITIONS

Patients who present with co-occurring mental illness and sleep disturbances will report either initial and/or terminal insomnia. Initial insomnia is usually indicative of an anxiety disorder such as generalized anxiety disorder, or an adjustment disorder with anxious mood. These patients have great difficulty falling asleep, but once they are asleep, they usually stay asleep throughout the night. Some patients present with middle insomnia (intermittent awakening); they fall asleep, but wake up periodically during the night. In addition, some have "early morning awakening" or terminal insomnia. These patients can usually fall asleep easily, but awaken around 3 or 4 A.M., and cannot get back to sleep. Most of these patients are likely to have a disorder with an affective component, such as major depression, schizoaffective disorder, dysthymia, or an adjustment disorder with depressed or mixed features.

Sometimes a patient presents with what appears to be a sleep-related disorder in addition to the types of poor sleeping patterns that are observed in the depressed or anxious patient. A primary care physician or neurologist should evaluate the patient for the presence of other dyssomnias or primary sleep disorders. The following list describes a few that may affect the patient:

1. *Obstructive Sleep Apnea (OSA).* This condition is troublesome for many patients. A milder form is called *upper airway resistance syndrome.* These conditions are much more common in overweight, middle-aged men, or patients with certain types of oropharyngeal and facial anatomies: The patient is unable to keep airways open during sleep, and the airway narrows or collapses leading to gasping or awakening throughout the night. Medications are usually not used here, and instead options include the continuous positive airway pressure machine or CPAP. This device splints the airway open and prevents airway narrowing during sleep. Surgery is an option for some, but it is rather drastic and only effective in about 50 percent of cases (Richert & Baran, 2003). Various mouth appliances have been designed to reposition the mandible, tongue, or both when sleeping. They have mixed, less-promising results and are usually only attempted by those with mild OSA.

2. *Sleep Bruxism.* Sleep-related teeth grinding is a parasomnia much more common among children, but it can be seen in adults during times of stress. In many cases psychotherapy and/or anxiety-reducing medications may improve this condition. A dentist may be consulted, and a mouth guard could be used to reduce the possibility of tooth damage or chronic headaches.

3. *Sleepwalking and Night Terrors.* These conditions are also typically seen in about 10 percent of children. Since they are usually outgrown, the use of medications such as benzodiazepines is not recommended for children or those patients with a history of substance dependence.

4. *Narcolepsy.* This condition consists of uncontrolled attacks of short-duration, restful sleep. The attacks are usually triggered by strong emotions such as laughter or anger. Since this condition may cause excessive daytime sleepiness, patients should receive counseling to assist with the stigma of the disorder and the perception that they are lazy or unmotivated. Short nap periods during the day, as well as consistent sleep/wake times are suggested.

Narcolepsy is typically treated with various psychostimulants such as methylphenidate (Ritalin), pemoline (Cylert), and now a newer medication modafinil (Provigil). Historically, stimulants have been used to reduce daytime sleepiness and sleep attacks, along with antidepressants to increase sleep quality. Modafinil is not considered a stimulant, and research suggests it may be less effective for narcoleptic patients, especially if they have been successfully treated with stimulants in the past (Brooks & Kushida, 2002). These researchers further state that some patients in Canada and France have responded to gamma-hydroxybutyrate (GHB), but it has not been approved for use in the United States. It received the name *date-rape drug* because it is abused as a party drug and often slipped into a beverage in the hope that someone taking the drug would be mentally impaired and willing to participate in sexual relations. Many patients often have impaired memory upon awakening. When taken for sleep disorders, GHB increases the quality of both REM and non-REM sleep cycles. Side effects of GHB include excessive grogginess and mental confusion before the drug wears off. The clinician needs to watch for signs of tolerance or dependency with stimulants used in the treatment of narcolepsy.

5. *Restless Legs Syndrome (RLS) and Periodic Leg Movement Disorder (PLMD).* These conditions often occur together, but they are distinct entities. Restless legs syndrome usually occurs in the evening and throughout the night. Patients complain of feeling restless or jittery and may not be able to relax. They often report that this feeling starts deep within their legs, and they often move or tap their feet to gain relief. Periodic leg movement disorder, which was previously known as nocturnal myoclonus, can cause sleep fragmentation and daytime sleepiness. With this disorder, the legs often jerk every few seconds, and this movement can increase in intensity to a point where sleep is seriously disturbed.

Treatment for both disorders involves either the use of benzodiazepines such as clonazepam (Klonopin) or the use of dopaminergic agents such as levodopa/carbidopa (Sinemet) or pramipexole (Mirapex). In severe cases, opioids may be considered. Research has shown that some patients with PLMD have iron, vitamin B_{12}, and folate deficiencies, so complete blood counts with differential should be ordered and evaluated (Richert & Baran, 2003).

In all cases of serious sleep disturbances, the clinician should order a complete sleep study or nocturnal polysomnogram (NPSG). This study is conducted at night in a sleep laboratory under the supervision of a neurologist or a sleep specialist. It involves recording multiple neurophysiologic and respiratory parameters during a patient's typical sleep period (often at night). Data are recorded from several places on the body including the following:

electroencephalogram (EEG) or brain-wave activity

electrocardiogram (EKG) and pulse

facial muscle movement

leg muscle movement

respiratory effort (chest and abdominal wall excursion)

oxygen saturation and carbon dioxide output

With the NPSG information, the clinician can more easily pinpoint the causes of various sleep disturbances and institute the appropriate treatment plan.

Before prescribing professionals consider medication, they should also determine if the sleep problem is chronic or brief in nature. Having occasional sleepless nights might be due to transient stress, poor sleeping environments, or lifestyle incompatibilities. Patients should be instructed in ways to improve their environments and make necessary lifestyle changes to reduce the frequency and intensity of these episodes. Most professionals would probably agree that occasional sleeplessness could be addressed with counseling or therapy sessions. If the patient is concerned about taking a prescription sleep medication, the clinician can suggest over-the-counter sleep aids such as Nidol, Sominex, Tylenol PM, or even Benadryl (brand of diphenhydramine).

BEHAVIORAL TECHNIQUES FOR TREATING SLEEP DISORDERS

Behavioral approaches such as relaxation training and biofeedback may be helpful in teaching patients ways to manage their sleep disturbances. While these techniques typically take longer to learn and do not offer immediate relief, they have been shown to have lasting effects that patients can employ long after medications have been discontinued (Doghramji, 2003). Many professionals use these behavioral techniques along with various medications for both immediate and lasting relief. All patients with sleep disturbances should consider these sleep-hygiene tips:

1. Reduce or eliminate the use of nicotine, alcohol, caffeine, or other stimulating substances, except those suggested by a health-care provider.

2. Try to maintain a regular sleep-wake cycle, that is, sleep and rise at the same time each day.

3. Avoid napping during the day unless advised to do so.

4. Use the bed only for sleeping and sex, not for thinking, working, reading, or watching TV.

5. Try to relax and unwind an hour before going to bed.

6. Try not to go to bed hungry; a light snack is permissible an hour before bed.

7. If you cannot sleep, don't lie there staring at the clock. Get up, read, watch TV, or engage in a nonstimulating activity in another room until you are tired.

8. Often moderate exercise during the day, or light exercise, such as walking an hour or so before bed, helps you to feel tired and sleep better.

9. A warm bath before bed helps to relax sore muscles and induce sleep.

10. Make a list two hours before bed of all activities you need to accomplish the next day. This will reduce the need to dwell on them while you are trying to relax and sleep.

11. Counseling or psychotherapy helps identify issues and reduce stress associated with sleep disturbances. Professionals can assist patients with coping skills and relaxation training.

12. Adjust temperature and noise and light levels in the room before you retire.

PHARMACOLOGY FOR SLEEP DISORDERS

Sedative-hypnotics are indicated in the treatment of most sleep disturbances. If the sleep disturbance is intermittent or temporary, these agents can be used safely for the short run without much concern for tolerance and dependence. If the patient appears to have a chronic problem, however, a careful examination must be made by the professional to evaluate the efficacy of using these medications for the long term, especially with patients who have a history of substance abuse or affective disorders. Except where indicated, patients should not use these medications, especially the benzodiazepines, for more than two to three weeks. Adequate evaluation and diagnosis should indicate the best course of action, which may include, a sleep study, physical examination, and psychotherapy where helpful.

In determining the best type of medication to use, half-life and onset of action are key points to consider. Sedating antidepressants may be helpful especially when the patient has an affective disorder (see Chapter 5). Most of these medications, however, also increase anticholinergic side effects such as weight gain, daytime drowsiness, dizziness, and orthostatic hypotension. Medications such as zaleplon (Sonata) have a rapid onset, but may wear off before the patient has had adequate sleep. See Table 11.1 for a list of medications used in the treatment of sleep disturbances.

Eszopiclone was approved by the FDA early in 2005 as a new treatment for insomnia. This novel, nonbenzodiazepine sleep aid marketed under the trade name of Lunesta is indicated for patients with both initial insomnia and those who have trouble sleeping through the night. Doses of 1–2 mg before bedtime are indicated for patients who have trouble falling asleep, while higher doses of 2–3 mg are indicated for those with sleep maintenance difficulty. The FDA approved eszopiclone for both short- and long-term treatment of insomnia, because it may pose less of an abuse and tolerance risk. It should be available for patient distribution in the summer of 2005.

Barbiturates such as amobarbital (Amytal), phenobarbital (Nembutal), and secobarbital (Seconal) will cause sedation and have been used in the past to treat insomnia; however, they are not used much today because they have a narrow therapeutic index, a high potential for abuse, and may interfere with normal sleep cycles.

Melatonin is an endogenous chemical produced in the pineal glad. The levels of melatonin reduce with age and may be further depleted if the patient regularly uses aspirin or ibuprofen. Various studies have demonstrated that taking 0.5–3 mg/day of melatonin may reduce the effects of insomnia due to jet lag and shift changes, but side effects include daytime drowsiness, cognitive slowing, and possibly, an increase in depression over time (Oxenkrug & Requintina, 2003).

TABLE 11.1 Medications Used in Treating Sleep Disturbances

TRADE NAME	GENERIC NAME	TYPICAL DOSE (MG/DAY)	ONSET OF ACTION
Benzodiazepines			
Dalmane	flurazepam	15–30	Rapid
Doral	quazepam	7.5–15	Rapid
Halcion	triazolam	0.125–0.25	Rapid
Prosom	estazolam	2–4	Rapid
Restoril	temazepam	15–30	Intermediate
Imidazopyridine			
Ambien	zolpidem	5–10	Rapid
Pyrazolopyrimidine			
Sonata	zaleplon	10–20	Rapid
Other			
Lunesta	eszopiclone	2–3	Rapid

Diphenhydramine (Benadryl) or other antihistamine hypnotics may be used to reduce problematic intermittent insomnia. A diphenhydramine dose of 25–50 mg/day is recommended, but like most sleep medications, should not be taken long term, as rebound insomnia may occur. Anticholinergic side effects are of course probable with these medications.

HOLISTIC TREATMENTS

The use of various holistic remedies have mixed results. These remedies may include substances like kava, which was used by the peoples of the South Pacific for thousands of years. Its action is similar to a sedative-hypnotic, because it appears to bind at the GABA receptors. Animal studies have shown that kava acts much like a benzodiazepine (Julien, 2001). More recently, the FDA, scientists, and others promoting holistic health have stated that kava may increase the risk of liver damage with prolonged use.

Valerian or valerian root has historically been used as a mild sedative, anxiolytic, and antidepressant. Its action is not well understood, but since GABA itself is a component of valerian, scientist and holistic advocates believe that valerian is a source of naturally occurring GABA. However, since GABA crosses the blood-brain barrier poorly, valerian is an unlikely source of GABA that would affect the central nervous system. Since valerian causes sedation, it should be used with caution by those taking other sedating medications. Valerian contains quercitin, a substance that inhibits the liver cytochrome enzymatic pathway CYP1A2. This inhibiting action could result in other significant drug interactions (Julien, 2001; Tyler, 1993).

As with all sedative-hypnotic treatments, the clinician must take great caution to correctly identify the type and nature of a patient's sleep difficulties. If medications are used, patients must be educated about typical side effects. Clinicians must use sedating medications with caution when prescribing them for elderly patients who often become disoriented during the night and might fall and injure themselves. Patients with a substance-abuse history should be carefully screened for stimulant-abuse potential and for the potential of excessive use of benzodiazepines.

..... ━━━━━━━━━━━━━━━━━━━━━━━━━━━━━

CHAPTER TWELVE

TREATMENT OF PERSONALITY DISORDERS

While there are technically no FDA approved medications for treating personality disorders, this chapter explores some common helpful medications or combinations of medications used in day-to-day practice for symptom reduction and control.

Topics to be addressed include the following:

- Use of medications for personality disorders
- Tailoring medications to symptom clusters
- Other concepts to consider

USE OF MEDICATIONS FOR PERSONALITY DISORDERS

Historically, psychotherapy has been the mainstay of treatment for Axis II syndromes, as opposed to pharmacotherapy which has been the primary therapeutic method for the majority of Axis I disorders. Medication treatment for personality disorders is a fairly new phenomenon in the field of psychopharmacology. Reich (2002) reports that epidemiological studies have consistently estimated that 10 percent of the population of the United States have a personality disorder. Other researchers have noted a prevalence rate for these disorders in the general population of up to 23 percent (Sadock & Sadock, 2000). Clinicians once believed that the use of medications in the treatment of personality disorders was counterproductive, because it would interfere with the psychotherapy. Today, both psychotherapy and psychopharmacological treatments are important considerations and used together.

Most types of psychotherapy have been used in the treatment of personality disorders. Each school of thought provides some understanding of behavior and method of intervention; however, the different schools are not mutually exclusive because they tend to overlap and complement one another. Numerous forms of psychotherapy have been tried including dynamic, behavioral, cognitive, supportive, and dialectical. As a general rule, the best way to approach these patients is to use combinations of various orientations. The emphasis should be on teamwork (i.e., doing something *with* the patient, not *to* the patient).

Research evidence suggests that personality disorders are a biopsychosocial entity caused by complex interactions of psychosocial and biological factors. For example, Livesley (2000) notes that twin studies indicate that personality disorder traits are genetically linked about 40 to 60 percent of the time. The variance is accounted for by specific environmental factors. When reviewing available information on twin studies, adoption studies, twins reared apart, and molecular genetics, researchers found significant evidence that antisocial and aggressive behaviors have genetic influences. Keep in mind that genetic processes need an environment in which to become expressed. Environmental stressors may turn genetic influences on and off across the life span (Raine, 2002). According to Kaylor (1999), impulsive and violent behavior may stem from brain dysfunction or damage secondary to head trauma, toxic chemical substances, trace elements in hair, focal lesions of the temporal lobe, low-serotonin levels, or other serotonergic dysfunction. These complicated interactions between nature and nurture will continue to be the focus of attention for many years to come.

Before considering pharmacotherapy for personality disorders, the clinician must obtain a comprehensive assessment (see Chapter 4 for details). Obtaining a complete psychiatric and medication history is not only important, but crucial. Target symptoms and their response to the pharmacotherapy, rather than treating the diagnosis, are the main focus. With the patient's permission, an interview with family members would be helpful in making a personality disorder diagnosis. An assessment of substance abuse or dependence is important and may mimic diagnostic symptoms of a personality disorder. Comorbidity also exists with respect to chemical dependency and personality disorders in a subset of the population. Family history is also valuable and may suggest the existence of biological vulnerabilities for mood disorders, drug and alcohol abuse, and perhaps personality disorders. Furthermore, endocrine, neurological, rheumatological, and metabolic disturbances may present as psychiatric illnesses, including personality or character disorders. Medications prescribed for these medical conditions may have cognitive, behavioral, or affective consequences. Laboratory evaluation, appropriate neuroimaging studies, and electroencephalogram (EEG) may be necessary in the evaluation to rule out confusing medical symptomatology.

TAILORING MEDICATIONS TO SYMPTOM CLUSTERS

First of all, clinicians need to know that are no FDA-approved medications for use in personality disorders. With the exception of avoidant personality disorder, there are no specific drugs for specific disorders. Then what are clinicians doing? They are basically treating comorbid Axis I diagnoses and personality disorder *traits*. Their goal is to find medications that they can appropriately use to treat the individual array of symptoms with which a patient presents. Although combinations of various classes of medications may be useful, clinicians should be mindful of polypharmacy also.

Most experts have defined three different symptom clusters, which prove to be useful. The clusters are as follows:

1. Paranoid, eccentric, thought disorder, dissociative cluster

2. Impulsive, depressive, angry, labile cluster

3. Anxious, inhibited, avoidant behavior cluster

This theoretical construct helps clinicians determine pharmacological treatment options. The three categories generally correspond to the DSM-IV-TR Personality Disorder Clusters A, B, and C. Each cluster will be considered and some recommendations for treatment will be made.

1. The paranoid, eccentric, thought disorder, dissociative cluster involves psychotic symptoms and a thought disorder that are theoretically on the mild end of the spectrum. Schizotypal personality disorder is a good example of this category. The treatment of choice would be an atypical antipsychotic medication because of the mild psychotic symptoms. As noted in Chapter 8, risperidone (Risperdal) is probably the best place to start; lower dosages are preferred. Reich (2002) recommends using about one-quarter to one-half of the usual dose that clinicians would use for other schizophrenic-related disorders. If the first antipsychotic fails, the clinician should then try a second atypical agent like olanzepine (Zyprexa) or quetiapine (Seroquel). Typical antipsychotics are not recommended because of the risk of tardive dyskinesia.

2. The impulsive, depressive, angry, labile cluster corresponds to Cluster B in the DSM-IV-TR. Impulsivity, aggression, mood lability, self-destructiveness, and suicidality are the main symptoms in this group. Although these symptoms are most commonly found in borderline personality disorder, they may occur in other forms in the other Cluster B diagnoses. For example, impulsivity and aggression in antisocial personality may present as lying, stealing, and destruction of property. Patients with these symptoms have a major disregard for social norms. In histrionic personality, low-frustration tolerance would correlate with this impulsivity and aggressiveness; narcissistic rage expressed in response to criticism would be a good example in that disorder.

With respect to medications, an SSRI antidepressant would be the most logical place to start. It should be titrated upward as tolerated to high doses, which are the doses used in obsessive-compulsive disorder. If one SSRI fails, try another. If the patient has a partial response to an SSRI, the clinician might consider augmenting with an atypical antipsychotic or a mood stabilizer. Some clinicians may use gabapentin (Neurontin) for anxiety, impulsivity, and sedation in these types of patients. They may use naltrexone (Revia), an opiate antagonist, if self-harming behaviors are prominent. As noted previously, combinations of medications may be the most useful.

3. The anxious, inhibited, avoidant behavior cluster may be manifested by shyness, diminished ability to function or use opportunities, rejection sensitivity, avoidant behaviors, and anxiety. Initially, an SSRI would be the treatment of choice. A second SSRI should be tried if the first one fails. With these patients, the clinician could consider a long-acting benzodiazepine such as clonazepam (Klonopin) as an adjunctive treatment option. Other considerations for treatment would be atypical antipsychotics, buspirone (Buspar), gabapentin, and perhaps beta-blockers. Some clinicians still use MAOIs to help

reduce isolative behaviors and rejection sensitivity. However, their use has declined since the introduction of medications with safer side-effect profiles. If patients have a history of substance abuse, remember to avoid benzodiazepines due to their addictive nature.

OTHER CONCEPTS TO CONSIDER

The duration of medication treatment with personality disorders is debatable. Treatment trials should last for at least four to six weeks to determine the drug's effectiveness (i.e., adequate trial). Although no patient should be on a medication longer than necessary, the clinician should be mindful that character issues are long term and chronic. If a drug or combination of drugs improves the patient symptomatically and has an acceptable low level of side effects, long-term treatment can be justified.

Personality traits and disorders are best conceptualized on a continuum. Hopefully, future research will illuminate the role of biological, psychological, and social factors in each personality disorder. Clinicians may then focus on primary prevention rather than treating the chronic sequelae of these illnesses.

■ ■ ■ ■ ■

CHAPTER THIRTEEN

TREATMENT OF CHEMICAL DEPENDENCY AND CO-OCCURRING CONDITIONS

This chapter looks at treatment considerations for people with co-occurring substance-abuse conditions. The dopamine hypothesis and relevant treatment issues are explored with helpful diagnostic instruments and pharmacological suggestions for each substance of concern.

Topics to be addressed include the following:

- Co-occurring conditions
- The dopamine hypothesis
- Treatment issues
- Assessment instruments and strategies
- Treatment phases and goals
- Psychopharmacology for dually-diagnosed patients
- Summary and treatment reminders

CO-OCCURRING CONDITIONS

For many patients presenting with various Axis I conditions, clinicians also observe the use and abuse of various substances. These substances may include alcohol and various other illegal drugs but may also include the abuse of prescription medications. The use of a substance, even to alter mood or the patient's physical state, is not necessarily problematic unless patients experience detrimental effects on their social and occupational functioning. Clinicians should try to examine the nature and intensity of drug use to determine if patients are compulsive in their use patterns and appear to have little control over the conditions and amounts used. Here the clinician is concerned with the following issues:

1. *Loss of control* (cannot stop or limit drug use)

2. T*olerance,* or the need to use more and more of the substance to avoid *withdrawal* or to maintain a desired state

3. *Impairment in functioning* such as failure to work or keep other life obligations

The clinician needs to evaluate these areas even if the patient meets full criteria for a singular diagnosis of substance abuse or dependence per the DSM-IV-TR.

Research into the use patterns of patients with co-occurring conditions indicates that substance abuse is a problem for about 61 percent of those with bipolar disorder, 47 percent of those with schizophrenia, 39 percent of those with personality disorders, 33 percent of those with obsessive-compulsive disorder, and 32 percent of those with an affective disorder (Reiger, et al 1990). It is not surprising to learn that the majority of patients who have been treated for a substance-abuse condition also meet criteria for another Axis I and/or Axis II diagnosis.

Although attempting to determine which condition came first may be nearly impossible, the clinician who can obtain a good history from the patient or the family may be able to accomplish this task. The clinician should consider the questions: In the absence of a family or personal history of mental illness, did the patient develop depression after years of abusing alcohol or drugs? After years of struggling with anxiety and panic, did the patient come to realize that drinking had a calmative effect and reduced the number of panic attacks? Did the ADHD teenager start abusing caffeine and speed once he noticed that it allowed him to relax and concentrate?

In patients with an existing Axis I and/or Axis II disorder, a co-occurring or dual-occurring substance abuse and mental illness disorder exists when the use of substances exceeds social use. For these patients, chemical-dependency treatment or detoxification (detox) may be needed. Determining the type and scope of treatment is based largely on the nature and intensity of the presenting problems and the particular treatment philosophy employed in the treatment setting.

Some researchers believe that chemical addiction is not simply a direct effect of the drug on the brain, but rather a pathological relationship that a person has with the drug (Schneider & Irons, 2001). Milkman (1987) and his colleagues found that *drugs and behaviors* can have addictive effects on the brain. When people pursue gratification, they experience three basic types of neurochemical responses: arousal, satiation, or an increase in preoccupation of the desired object (fantasy). *Arousal* is accompanied by an increase in dopamine and norepinephrine, satiation with GABA, and fantasy with serotonin. Typically, people seeking arousal use drugs that increase arousal (cocaine or amphetamines), or they engage in high-risk behaviors such as gambling; both activities increase dopamine and norepinephrine. A sedation and/or *satiation* response could be achieved with excessive food consumption, television watching, video games, or drugs like benzodiazepines or alcohol. *Fantasy* is often the core issue in sexual addiction. Researchers believe that when a person is addicted, the addiction is in fact to a *set of behaviors involving a drug or an activity.* The behavioral activities themselves can produce chemical changes in the brain similar to those produced by any exogenous drug.

THE DOPAMINE HYPOTHESIS

Most drugs of abuse, including cigarettes, increase the concentration of dopamine in the nucleus accumbens and the mesolimbic system (the brain's reward centers). Over-stimulation exhausts the dopamine system and causes the brain to reduce both the amount of dopamine available and the receptor sites they bind with. Most abusers start out seeking the high that comes from drug use, later they use drugs to avoid withdrawal. In withdrawal they experience dysphoria and depression because of an increase in dopamine 3 receptor sites that are craving or looking for dopamine. Much of the psychopharmacology used in the treatment of patients with co-occurring conditions attempts to address depression, anxiety, and craving to increase the patient's chances of a sustained recovery.

TREATMENT ISSUES

While most treatment centers (and the general public) adhere to a zero-tolerance model that emphasizes total abstinence, some researchers believe that the patient could learn harm-reduction techniques leading to nonsymptomatic, responsible use (Marlatt & Witkiewitz, 2002). These researchers further mention that empirical studies have demonstrated that harm-reduction approaches to alcohol are at least as effective as abstinence-based treatment approaches at reducing alcohol consumption and alcohol related consequences.

As mentioned earlier, treatment centers tend to have their own unique philosophies about detox and recovery. Some centers adhere to the traditional moral model, often utilizing some type of 12-step approach. Others employ more of a *rational-recovery* viewpoint, assuming that patients may not buy into a spiritual or religious reason for their use or recovery. Still other centers consider the disease model that assumes complete abstinence with no return to nonproblematic or social use of any kind.

A good treatment center takes *all* modalities into consideration. It neither assumes that the patient is self-medicating an Axis I or II condition, nor does it assume that all of the patient's behaviors are caused by drug use. The center also does not assume that all patients have "chemically addicted brains" and can never use a drug again. The center treats both co-occurring issues together and watches to see if after treatment, a singular condition reemerges to be treated more aggressively.

ASSESSMENT INSTRUMENTS AND STRATEGIES

Many evaluation instruments can be used to assess client readiness for recovery and levels of resistance. The Michigan Alcohol Screening Test (MAST) is a short, 24-item questionnaire in a yes/no format that detects the presence and extent of drinking. A shorter, 13-item version is also available. The Substance Abuse Subtle Screening Inventory (SASSI-3) is a 67-item instrument that measures issues like openness, chemical dependency predisposition, and defensiveness. The Substance Abuse Life Circumstance Evaluation (SALCE) contains 98 items and may be helpful in identifying triggers for relapse, for example, the patient's levels of stress. The MacAndrew Alcoholism Scale of the MMPI-2 is helpful in identifying the potential for drug or alcohol abuse in a patient. The Substance Abuse Problem Checklist consists of 377 items and examines problematic areas such as treatment motivation, health problems, personality issues, social relationships, job problems, leisure issues, legal issues, and spirituality. This checklist is helpful in assessing patients who have co-occurring personality disorders and social concerns.

For many clinicians, who do not work in chemical dependency settings, substance-abuse screening is often determined simply from historical information. In this case, using the CAGE questionnaire is helpful:

1. Have you ever felt that you should *Cut* down on your drinking (or drug use)?

2. Have people *Annoyed* you by criticizing your drinking (or drug use)?

3. Have you ever felt bad or *Guilty* about your drinking (or drug use)?

4. Have you ever had a drink (or used drugs) first thing in the morning (an *Eye* opener) to steady your nerves or get rid of a hangover?

TREATMENT PHASES AND GOALS

In most treatment centers, treatment is achieved in a series of steps or phases of treatment. A typical first phase involves a complete assessment of the patient and his or her situation. Here the clinician obtains the nature and patterns of drug use as well as related emotions. A detailed history is taken including the types of drugs abused, dates of use, attempts at treatment, relevant legal or medical problems, and the extent of financial hardships caused by their condition. In determining the nature of drug use, the clinician needs to inquire about the intensity and frequency of the patient's use of drugs. Patients who use drugs on a steady basis may exhibit more antisocial tendencies; patients who are more like binge users are more likely to use drugs for self-medication or social lubrication reasons. The clinician will find it helpful to interview spouses, partners, and other family members to learn how they view the patient and his or her level of functioning.

In the second phase of treatment, the clinician attempts to determine the special needs of the dually-diagnosed patient. The following questions guide this effort.

1. Does the patient need medically supervised detox?

2. Does the patient need psychotropic medication or a psychiatric evaluation?

3. Does the patient need inpatient observation based on the patient's behaviors or threats?

4. What is the patient's level of resistance?

5. What is the patient's potential for relapse?

6. What, if any, are the environmental issues that affect treatment (i.e., childcare, work, finances, spousal abuse, codependency, enabling issues, etc.)?

In phase three of treatment, the clincian examines the need for using various medications in the treatment of the patient with co-occurring concerns. The clinician should carefully weigh the use of psychotropic medications. In most cases only antidepressants and appropriate antipsychotics should be considered. The use of pain medications and/or anxiolytics should be avoided, except during the initial stages of detox and only when the clinician determines that their use outweighs the risks (Sattar & Bhatia, 2003).

PSYCHOPHARMACOLOGY FOR DUALLY-DIAGNOSED PATIENTS

This section describes medications and various other substances that are used in the treatment of dually-diagnosed patients for alchohol, opioid, and cocaine dependence and other addictions.

Alcohol Dependence

1. Disulfiram (Antabuse) is used as a form of "aversion" therapy, because it causes a very unpleasant chemical reaction when patients who use it drink alcohol. Typically, the enzyme acetaldehyde dehydrogenase converts acetaldehyde to harmless acetate, but disulfiram interferes with this process and allows toxic acetaldehyde to accumulate when alcohol is consumed causing nausea, sweating, and rapid pulse. While not life threatening to most patients, this medication is not indicated for those who have serious health concerns or for cardiovascular patients. The typical dose is 125–250 mg/day, but doses of up to 500 mg/day may be considered. The clinician should know that this medication can stay in a patient's system for several days after discontinuance, so drug holidays may still lead to chemical reactions in patients who "fall off the wagon." For this reason, disulfiram is most helpful for binge drinkers trying to maintain sobriety. While most patients tolerate this medication without difficulty, some complain of mild gastrointestinal upset. The clinician might suggest taking the medication with food to avoid these side effects.

Some treatment centers request that the medication be given by a family member to assure compliance. When the medication is obtained from the pharmacy, the pharmacist will give the patient some other instructions. For example, if disulfiram is used with any alcohol-containing product such as aftershave, mouthwash, or rubbing alcohol, unpleasant rashes or other side effects can result.

2. Naltrexone (Revia) mimics the action of naturally occurring opioid neurotransmitters in the brain. In animal studies, when opioid antagonists were administered, the animals consumed less alcohol. In human studies, patients reduced their levels of

drinking and reported prolonged abstinence. The typical daily dose of naltrexone is 50 mg/day. Side effects may include sedation, nausea, and liver dysfunction. This medication is not indicated for patients with compromised liver functioning, because higher doses of naltrexone have been associated with liver toxicity. This medication is best suited for patients who are early in recovery and who are steady users.

3. Nalmefene (Revex), at the writing of this text, was not indicated for use in chemically dependent patients. However, the drug is FDA approved for complete or partial reversal of opioid drug effects and is used primarily in the field of anesthesia. As with naltrexone, endogenous opioid brain circuits are blocked, thus blocking the dopamine-mediated euphoria. Nalmefene is a mu-opioid antagonist with fewer side effects and a longer half-life than naltrexone.

4. Acamprosate (Campral) was approved by the FDA in 2004 for use in patients with alcohol dependence. It has been used in Europe for many years. Although the mechanism of action is unknown, researchers believe that acamprosate may facilitate the calming action of GABA at its receptors, while inhibiting glutamate (an excitatory neurotransmitter). Acamprosate may reduce the hyperexcitability associated with alcohol withdrawal and craving. The typical dose is approximately 2000 mg/day.

The use of benzodiazepines is typically reserved for detox settings and not recommended for maintenance because of the possibility of developing dependence. Some clinicians find that SSRIs, such as fluoxetine (Prozac) or sertraline (Zoloft), are helpful and may reduce alcohol use, but only in patients with a co-occurring affective disorder. Some research suggests that ondansetron (Zofran), which is used to reduce nausea in chemotherapy cancer patients and bulimia nervosa patients, may help reduce carvings for both alcohol and methamphetamine (Psychopharmacology Update, 2003).

Opioid Dependence

1. Methadone (Dolophine) is a synthetic opiate that is taken orally (liquid). It produces a minimal high and sedation and has few side effects at therapeutic doses. While controversial, methadone-maintenance programs have helped many heroin users return to work and maintain family obligations. Typical methadone doses range from 20–200 mg/day, depending on the severity of the addiction.

2. L-alpha-acetyl-methadol or *l*ong *a*cting *a*nalog *m*ethadone (LAAM) has properties that are similar to methadone, but it has been shown to be superior to methadone in reducing intravenous drug use. Since it has a slower onset of action and a longer half-life, it can be administered only three times per week rather than daily like methadone. Typical doses of LAAM start at 20 mg, three times per week and may go up to 80 mg, three times per week. This medication may not be indicated for cardiac patients per FDA warnings.

3. Buprenorphine (Subutex) is a mixed, opioid agonist–antagonist used as an analgesic. In treatment centers, it is given sublingually at 2–4 mg/day and can be increased to 16 mg/day if needed. Advantages of buprenorphine include a milder withdrawal upon discontinuance and less potential for abuse, because the agonist effects are diminished at higher doses.

4. Naloxone (Narcan) is used to reverse the effects of an opioid overdose. While medications like naloxone act as antagonists and shorten withdrawal, they also cause the withdrawal to be rather intense. A procedure called *ultra-rapid detox* uses naloxone in combination with clonidine or other sedatives for a 24-hour detoxification. This medication is also available as a mixed compound with buprenorphine called Suboxone (buprenorphine/naloxone).

Cocaine Dependence

1. Tricyclic antidepressants like desipramine (Norpramin) have shown some promise in reducing cravings and improving abstinence associated with cocaine abuse, even when depression is not present.

2. Bromocriptine (Parlodel), amantadine (Symmetrel), and mazindol (Sanorex/ Mazanor) are dopamine agonists that are given to reduce craving and discomfort in the early stages of cocaine withdrawal. Typical doses are 0.125 mg every 4 hours.

3. Ibogain is derived from the root of the African iboga shrub. This botanical substance is an indole alkaloid that helps to mask cocaine and opioid withdrawal, but it is a potent hallucinogen with a potential for abuse. Ibogain was shown to reduce stimulant use in lab animals. It may have some promise as a treatment for stimulant abuse as well (Jullien, 2001). Typical doses range from 10–60 mg/day.

4. Methylphenidate (Ritalin) has been shown to reduce cocaine relapse, especially in patients with ADHD. Typical doses range from 15–60 mg/day (see Chapter 9 for details regarding its use).

5. Buprenorphine (Subutex) is a mixed, opioid agonist–antagonist used as an analgesic. In treatment centers, it is given sublingually at 2–4 mg/day and can be increased to 16 mg/day if needed. Advantages of buprenorphine include a milder withdrawal upon discontinuance and less potential for abuse, because the agonist effects are diminished at higher doses.

Other Types of Addiction

Bupropion (Wellbutrin SR/Zyban) has been FDA approved in the treatment of nicotine addiction. It has been shown to be more effective than nicotine replacement gums or patches in reducing relapse in smokers (Williams & Hughes, 2003). This result was found to be especially true when a co-occurring depression was present. Nicotine dependence has a high comorbidity not only with depression but with conduct disorder and ADHD as well.

Because SSRIs often reduce sexual appetite, they may offer some hope to people with sexual addiction and compulsivity. Sexual-addiction disorders often coexist with chemical dependency and frequently trigger relapse (Schneider & Irons, 2001). This research also mentions that as many as 70 percent of cocaine addicts are also sexually addicted, and as many as 76 percent of methamphetamine users consider themselves to be "sexually obsessed."

SUMMARY AND TREATMENT REMINDERS

In the fourth or final phase of treatment, the clinician assesses how the patient has progressed and the need for more attention to either the substance-abuse issue or the mental-health issue. Clinicians must keep in mind that when treating the primary mental-health diagnosis with medications, they are not compromising the patient's chemical dependency issues (i.e., treating an anxiety disorder with benzodiazepines in a patient with a history of alcohol dependence). In this situation, the clinician is likely to see abuse of the benzodiazepines. Another common example is the anxious patient who is trying to remain substance free and presents with a chief complaint of initial insomnia. The patient's physician gives the patient a sedative-hypnotic as a sleep aid only to learn months later that the patient has become dependent on them.

Clinicians also need to be sensitive with respect to patients that they refer to Alcoholics Anonymous (AA) and Narcotics Anonymous (NA) groups. Most of these groups have little tolerance for people with co-occurring conditions and are likely to hassle them for taking "other drugs" for their condition. The clinician needs to inquire about the group's composition and send patients only to groups that are sensitive to the medication issues.

Preventing a patient's relapse is the key to continued success, and reducing stress is the key to preventing relapse. "Booster" sessions and stress-reduction groups are excellent ideas. While relapse tends to happen in about 50 percent of all cases, clinicians should have a clear plan for resuming treatment without a heavy emphasis on failure that will allow patients to rework their program without shame and to strive for full recovery.

CHAPTER FOURTEEN

TREATMENT OF COMORBIDITY AND OTHER DISORDERS

This chapter examines the often complex role of comorbid conditions. All clinicians deal with patients who present with issues such as chronic pain, eating disorders and obesity, and, of course, disorders of impulse control, but few suggestions for treatment are presented in most psychopharmacology texts. Helpful pharmacological considerations are presented here with a rationale for symptom reduction.

Topics to be addressed include the following:

- Medical and psychiatric cormorbidity
- Chronic pain
- Eating disorders and obesity
- Impulse control disorders

Psychiatric disorders exist in real life, not in an isolated system, but rather within the context of other serious, medical and psychiatric diagnoses. Besides looking at the various medical and psychiatric comorbidities, in this chapter we consider other important psychiatric issues including chronic pain, eating disorders, obesity, and impulse-control disorders. Frequently, these diseases co-occur with multiple other medical illnesses. The common features that bind these topics together are the complexity and sometimes resistant nature of their treatment. According to Kroenke (2003), unexplained or multiple somatic symptoms are the leading cause of outpatient medical visits and also the predominant reason why patients with common mental disorders, such as anxiety and depression, initially present in primary care.

MEDICAL AND PSYCHIATRIC COMORBIDITY

The complicated interaction between the mind and body may lead to disease processes that are more difficult to treat than individual illnesses themselves. According to Blazer, Steffens, and Busse (2004), depression has been shown to be a risk factor for declines in physical functioning; likewise, declines in physical functioning have been shown to be a risk factor for depression. Attention to psychiatric symptoms among medically ill patients has emerged in general medical settings over the last ten years or so. Kroenke (2003) reports that patients have at least a twofold greater risk of experiencing a depressive or anxiety disorder if they have a concomitant disease including cardiovascular disease, neurological disease, cancer, diabetes, HIV, and many other physical disorders. Psychiatric comorbidities are important factors that may increase the length of acute medical/surgical inpatient stays, the frequency of medical complications, and the overall mortality (Sadock & Sadock, 2000).

Depression often co-occurs with a variety of psychiatric and substance abuse/dependence disorders. When co-occurrence happens, the presence of both illnesses is frequently unrecognized and, unfortunately, leads to serious and unnecessary negative consequences for patients and families. According to Kupfer and Frank (2003), concurrent depression is present in 13 percent of patients with panic disorder. With respect to eating disorders, 50 to 75 percent of patients suffering from anorexia nervosa or bulimia nervosa have a lifetime history of major depressive disorder. These high levels of comorbid diagnoses with depression are also true for substance-abuse disorders (see Chapter 13). When Axis II disorders are considered, dysfunctional personality traits have a negative effect on the outcome of treatment of Axis I disorders (Reich, 2003).

When looking at concurrent medical disease, Lesperance, Frasure-Smith, and Talajic (1996) demonstrated that 40 to 65 percent of patients who have experienced a myocardial infarction suffer from depression. The point prevalence of major depression in patients with coronary artery disease is estimated at 17 to 22 percent; this prevalence is roughly twice that in primary care patients and three to four times the point prevalence in the population at large (Sadock & Sadock, 2000). In general practice, cancer patients suffer from depression about 25 percent of the time according to many experts. In patients with neurological diseases (e.g., stroke), researchers suggest that depression occurs in the range of 25 percent. Morbidity and mortality continue to increase in connection with the number of medical and/or psychiatric diagnoses (Kupfer & Frank, 2003).

Even in the medical-psychiatric comorbidity context, the treatment of the particular psychiatric diagnosis is very similar to the treatment of the psychiatric problem alone. For example, depression either alone or in the context of a comorbid medical condition should be treated similarly. However, the clinician should use the lowest-possible medication dose to treat the disorder, especially when multiple conditions are being treated with many different pharmacotherapies. Communication between the various prescribers treating the patient's co-occurring conditions is of utmost importance.

The field of psychosomatic medicine is a rapidly evolving and increasingly important area of study. Although beyond the scope of this chapter, significant connections exist between a patient's psychological status and various disease conditions. Current fields of study related to comorbidity include psychocardiology, psychoneuroimmunology, psychoneuroendocrinology, psycho-oncology, and functional gastrointestinal disorders.

CHRONIC PAIN

According to the International Association for the Study of Pain, pain is an unpleasant sensory and emotional experience associated with actual or potential tissue damage (Merskey, 1979). The emotional experience part of the definition was even noted by Freud in the 1890s (Strachey, 1953). Since pain is neither a purely physiological state nor a purely psychological one, treatment demands a comprehensive, integrated, multidisciplinary plan as well as clear communication of all findings to the patient. The clinician must keep in mind that there is no typical pain patient; individualized treatment is absolutely necessary.

Although many chronic-pain patients resist psychiatric help, a formal psychiatric consultation is important to clarify the medical diagnoses, screen for psychiatric diagnoses, and identify emotional influences that underlie or exacerbate primary pain. Chronic pain may be a presenting symptom of many of the following psychiatric diagnoses: major depression, generalized anxiety disorder, panic disorder, posttraumatic stress disorder, and substance abuse. Other less-common psychiatric diagnoses that may be present in the context of chronic pain include delusional disorders, chronic psychosis, somatoform disorders, and malingering. Furthermore, emotional influences that may affect the pain experience include unresolved grief; sexual or developmental conflicts; sexual, physical, or emotional abuse; anger at physicians; and even symbolic identification with a loved one (Mufson, 1999).

From the psychiatric perspective, treatment of chronic pain and its emotional components relies on medications and various forms of psychotherapy. Antidepressants are probably the most prescribed group of medications because of their effect on improving mood and decreasing anxiety. Tricyclic antidepressents are still widely used in this context not only for reasons already mentioned (see Chapter 5), but also for their noradrenergic effects that decrease neuropathic pain. Many pain physicians use amitriptyline (Elavil) in a 25 mg dose at bedtime to help decrease pain, improve sleep, and possibly improve mood. As a class, the SNRIs (serotonin- norepinephrine reuptake inhibitors) such as venlafaxine (Effexor) and duloxetine (Cymbalta) may be more effective than SSRIs at decreasing the somatic symptoms associated with depression and anxiety syndromes (Grothe, Scheckner, & Albano, 2004). Finally, Bischofs, Zelenka, and Sommer (2004) report that topiramate (Topamax), an anticonvulsant mood stabilizer, decreases neuropathic pain and improves mood lability.

Psychotherapeutic options for chronic-pain patients include individual, marital, and family therapy to address the underlying dynamic factors. Cognitive behavioral therapy, hypnosis, and biofeedback are probably the most useful and most practical ways to approach these complicated and challenging patients.

EATING DISORDERS AND OBESITY

The eating disorders are a complex group of illnesses that are heavily underpinned by psychopathology and are associated with significant medical consequences. These disorders primarily affect young women. Patients who suffer from anorexia nervosa and bulimia nervosa place extraordinary emphasis on weight, shape, and the pursuit of thinness. Most recently, binge-eating disorder, which is characterized by episodes of uncontrollable eating, has emerged as a diagnostic entity. Patients with eating disorders tend to have high rates of psychiatric comorbidity and medical complications (Pederson, Roerig, & Mitchell, 2003). Furthermore, obesity is discussed because of the prominent nature it plays in one's self-concept as well as societal views of beauty and attractiveness.

Anorexia Nervosa

Anorexia nervosa is characterized by patients' refusal to maintain a normal body weight along with their intense fear of gaining weight despite being underweight. According to Pederson, Roerig, and Mitchell (2003), the disorder can lead to serious medical consequences including osteoporosis, cardiac arrhythmias, and congestive heart failure. The estimates of comorbidity rates in eating disorder patients indicate that 50 to 75 percent of patients have comorbid depression, approximately 25 percent of patients have obsessive-compulsive disorder, and 42 to 75 percent of patients have a personality disorder (APA website, 2004).

Anorexia nervosa has two distinct phases of the illness: acute, underweight phase (usually inpatient) and the maintenance, weight-restored phase (usually outpatient). The two phases basically represent different biological entities in that the treatment options differ. In the acute phase of treatment with patients close to emaciation, the treatment plan largely focuses on inpatient care, medically supervised refeeding programs, dietary counseling, and individual, group, and family therapies. Medications play a more significant role in the maintenance, weight-restored phase of treatment. Although anorexia nervosa was defined as a diagnostic entity over a century ago, the absolute etiology underlying the disorder remains elusive (Pederson et.al, 2003; Mitchell, de Zwaan, & Roerig, 2003).

A large variety of compounds have been explored in treating anorexia nervosa including antidepressants, antipsychotics, antihistamines, narcotic antagonists, lithium, and zinc to name a few. Controlled medication trials in patients with anorexia nervosa are few in number; thus, optimal treatment has yet to be defined. Research has predominately focused on two drug groups: antidepressants and antipsychotics. Trials of TCAs and fluoxetine (Prozac) have not been shown to offer much benefit for the acute treatment phase. However, a controlled, outpatient maintenance trial suggests that patients randomized to fluoxetine gained more weight, had decreased core eating-disorder symptoms, and displayed more improvement in mood symptoms compared with the placebo group at the one-year endpoint (Kaye, Nagata, & Weltzin, 2001). Both in terms of stimulating weight gain and in reducing delusional thoughts about food, weight, and shape, pilot studies and case reports have described successful use of atypical antipsychotics such as olanzepine (Zyprexa) and risperidone (Risperdal) in anorexia nervosa patients.

Bulimia Nervosa

In contrast to anorexia nervosa, which is relatively rare, bulimia nervosa is more prevalent and affects about 1 to 3 percent of adolescent and young-adult females. Bulimia nervosa patients place great emphasis on body weight and shape, but unlike anorexia nervosa patients, they usually fall within a normal weight range. This disorder is characterized by binge-eating episodes and associated inappropriate compensatory behaviors aimed at preventing weight gain. Medical consequences of bulimia nervosa include dental complications (permanent loss of tooth enamel, increased frequency of caries, and parotid gland swelling), amenorrhea, electrolyte abnormalities, esophageal tears, gastric rupture, and cardiac arrhythmias. The last three medical conditions may be fatal. As with anorexia nervosa, bulimia nervosa patients have high rates of comorbid psychopathology: about 50 percent have a lifetime diagnosis of depression, about 25 percent have a lifetime diagnosis of substance abuse or dependence, and about 40 percent have a personality disorder (Agras, 2001). The cause of bulimia is uncertain, but mounting evidence suggests that genetic factors play an important role (Bulik, Devlin, & Bacanu, 2003). Disturbances in serotonergic systems may play a role in causing bulimia because of the involvement of serotonin in the regulation of food intake. Cultural attitudes toward standards of physical attractiveness are also believed to contribute to causation (Mehler, 2003).

Bulimia nervosa has been more extensively studied than anorexia. Pharmacotherapy with antidepressants results in significant reductions in target eating behaviors such as binge eating and vomiting and associated mood or anxiety disorders. The only FDA-approved treatment for bulimia nervosa is fluoxetine (Prozac) in the dosage range of 60–80 mg/d. Furthermore, studies have consistently shown that cognitive-behavior therapy (CBT) is the first-line treatment of choice when it is available. Although CBT alone is superior to medication treatment alone, most experts would consider the use of CBT plus an antidepressant to be more effective than either treatment alone (Mitchell, Peterson, Myers & Wonderlich, 2001). Other medications studied that may be useful in treating bulimia include odansetron (Zofran), a 5-HT$_3$ antagonist, and topiramate (Topamax), an anticonvulsant mood stabilizer. Further studies involving nonantidepressants are needed to establish efficacy.

Binge-Eating Disorder

Finally, binge-eating disorder (BED) is characterized by binge-eating patterns similar to bulimic patients without compensatory weight-loss behaviors such as purging episodes or overexercising. The estimated prevalence of BED is 1.5 to 2 percent in the general population. When looking at obese populations such as those seeking weight-loss assistance programs, the prevalence of BED increases to 8 to 19 percent (Devlin, 2002). In bariatric surgery programs, Wadden, Sarwer, and Womble (2001) report that approximately 25 percent of the individuals may have BED.

Treatment efforts for BED have included TCAs, SSRIs, anticonvulsants, and antiobesity medications. Unlike the information available for bulimia nervosa, pharmacological data for treatment of BED are much more preliminary. Cognitive-behavior therapy appears to be more efficacious than SSRIs in about half of the controlled trials. More recently, research has focused on topiramate (Topamax) and sibutramine (Meridia) as future possibilities for decreasing the psychopathology and promoting weight loss (Pederson et.al. 2003). Sibutramine (Meridia) is an SNRI like venlafaxine (Effexor) and duloxetine (Cymbalta).

Obesity

Obesity is another prevalent disease that affects over 60 million Americans today. Approximately 64 percent of adult Americans are categorized as being overweight (body mass index (BMI) of 25–29.9 kg/m^2) or obese (BMI more than 30 kg/m^2). Obesity is associated with increased mortality and comorbidities such as hypertension, hyperglycemia, dyslipidemia, coronary artery disease, and certain cancers. The suggested goal for weight loss is to achieve a 10 percent weight reduction in six months through lifestyle changes. If lifestyle changes alone are not effective, then pharmacotherapy may be indicated (American Obesity Association website, 2004).

Over the last few years, fenfluramine (Pondimin), dexfenfluramine (Redux), and phenylpropanolamine (an ingredient in over-the-counter nasal decongestants and weight-control drugs) have been withdrawn by the FDA because of severe adverse effects. The only medications approved by the FDA as anorectics are the following: phentermine (Adipex-P/Ionamin), sibutramine (Meridia), and orlistat (Xenical). According to Campbell and Mathys (2001), phentermine has been shown to cause 5 to 15 percent weight loss if given daily or intermittently. The limiting factor with this medication is that it is only approved for short-term use and tolerance often develops.

Sibutramine acts as an SNRI and increases both norepinephrine and serotonin levels. However, it should not be prescribed with most antidepressants because of the risk of increased norepinephrine and serotonin levels. In patients with cardiovascular disease, sibutramine is contraindicated due to the possibility of hypertension and tachycardia.

Orlistat (Xenical) works as a reversible inhibitor of lipases in the gastrointestinal tract; these inactivated enzymes are unavailable to hydrolyze dietary fat, and thus the fats are not absorbed. Orlistat has an advantage over the other medications in that it is not absorbed systemically, and it may have cholesterol-lowering effects in some patients. Unfortunately, orlistat is less desirable in some patients due to the high incidence of gastrointestinal side effects, and it must be given three times daily with meals.

Other antiobesity drugs are being studied including, but not limited to, nutrients, neuropeptides, mazindol (Sanorex/Mazanor), antidepressants, anticonvulsants, growth hormone fragments, and so on. Due to the brevity of the discussion here, other treatments options have not been explored but include dietary therapy, physical activity, behavior therapy, combination therapy, and even bariatric surgery.

IMPULSE-CONTROL DISORDERS

The impulse-control disorders are characterized by the failure to resist an impulse, drive, or temptation to perform some act that is harmful to the patient or others. In most cases, the patient senses increasing tension or arousal prior to the act and experiences pleasure, gratification, or relief during or following the act. These disorders include kleptomania, pathological gambling, trichotillomania, pyromania, intermittent-explosive disorder, and the residual not otherwise specified category. Potential diagnoses such as compulsive buying and self-mutilation are appropriate examples of this

NOS category. Some researchers have proposed that these disorders of impulses be more specifically called *obsessive-compulsive spectrum disorders*, which might also include somatoform disorders, eating disorders, dissociative disorders, and some neurological disorders (e.g., Tourette's disorder).

In addition to the cognitive-behavioral strategies used with these disorders, successful psychopharmacological interventions have been described throughout the literature. For treating kleptomania, various serotonergic antidepressants including fluvoxamine (Luvox), fluoxetine (Prozac), clomipramine (Anafranil), amitriptyline (Elavil), imipramine (Tofranil), nortriptyline (Pamelor), and trazodone (Desyrel) have been used with some success (Sadock & Sadock, 2000). Mood stabilizers such as lithium, valproate (Depakote), and topiramate (Topamax) have been successful in some case studies (Dannon, 2003). As mentioned in Chapter 13, opioid-receptor antagonists such as naltrexone (Revia) have been used with the impulse-control disorders resulting in positive outcomes for some. Pathological gambling and trichotillomania have been treated similarly to kleptomania with the SSRIs, mood stabilizers, and opioid antagonists offering some success. Atypical antipsychotics such as risperidone (Risperdal) or olanzepine (Zyprexa) have also been attempted in some cases with a positive response. For intermittent-explosive disorder, research evidence suggests that mood stabilizers, atypical antipsychotics, beta-blockers, alpha-2 agonists, phenytoin (Dilantin), and serotonergic antidepressants may be useful (Olvera, 2002).

Although we have focused only on medical-psychiatric comorbidity, chronic pain, eating disorders, obesity, and impulse-control disorders, medications may be used with some effectiveness for many other psychiatric diagnoses. Most of these areas of study are based on small case reports or anecdotal evidence from busy clinicians.

CHAPTER FIFTEEN

CASE VIGNETTES: CHILDREN

NAPOLEON

Clinical History

Napoleon is a 9-year-old, Hispanic male with a four-year history of behavior problems consisting of hyperactivity, impulsivity, and incorrigibility. He presented to a community mental health clinic for evaluation and treatment. His mother reported that her son had always been extremely moody and had difficulty sitting still, paying attention in school, and following rules. The mother was getting to the point where she could not manage him anymore, and she may need to look into placement options because his behavior was uncontrollable. During the clinical interview, further details about Napoleon were obtained, including his extremely irritable moods, elevated or euphoric moods, grandiose ideas about the future, severe bouts of depression, distractibility, frequent use of profanity, and sexually inappropriate comments toward females. Napoleon's self-esteem seemed to correlate with his moods, as did his school performance. Napoleon also reported that when he was sad, he heard the voice of the devil who told him that he was no good and should die. On the other hand when his mood was "really good," Napoleon heard God's voice telling him that he was special.

Napoleon's mother reported that he had always been fairly healthy except for the use of an inhaler at times for his asthma. When asked about psychiatric family history, his mother reported that she had some mood swings when she was younger and was hospitalized on two occasions. Although she had taken medications, she was unable to recall the names of the medications or the diagnosis for which she had been treated. Napoleon's maternal grandfather was an alcoholic and went on intermittent binges.

Napoleon's mother recalled that her son had taken medications such as Ritalin and Dexedrine in the past, but they reduced his appetite without any therapeutic benefit. Napoleon has been disruptive in school and was frequently sent home for his bad behavior. However, he has gone weeks or months at a time without any behavioral problems in school.

Postcase Discussion and Diagnosis

Napoleon appears to have some symptoms consistent with ADHD as well as bipolar disorder. When his mother was questioned in more detail, further symptoms emerged, including periods of increased energy and hyperactivity, a decreased need for sleep, grandiose thoughts with hyperreligiosity, increased verbal output (nonpressured speech), and being easily distractible. Following these elevated moods, Napoleon would experience depressed periods characterized by hypersomnia, poor appetite, intermittent voices (mood congruent), low energy, sense of hopelessness, and anhedonia. Given the family's history of bipolar spectrum disorders (the mother's moodiness and the grandfather's binge drinking), Napoleon appears to have bipolar disorder NOS (296.80) and needs immediate treatment. Since suicidality is not present, treatment can be initiated in the outpatient setting with his mother's consent and support. Inpatient treatment may be necessary if Napoleon becomes a danger to himself, a danger to others, and/or unmanageable in the home for his mother.

Proposed Psychopharmacological Treatment

After an appropriate medical and psychiatric evaluation, Napoleon was started on lithium 150 mg twice daily with a plan to increase as tolerated to a dose of 600–900 mg/d. Lithium was chosen for its tolerability and effectiveness. When starting any psychotropic medication in children, parents must watch the child closely and monitor his or her moods on a daily basis. Prior to starting the lithium, appropriate laboratory testing was done and will be followed per typical protocols.

When Napoleon returned for a follow-up visit ten days later, he was feeling OK taking lithium, 600 mg/d. His mother reported that he had been doing much better. He was less impulsive and irritabile, his sleeping patterns improved, and his moods were more level or even. Napoleon and his mother agreed to proceed with outpatient medication management and to engage in psychotherapy to address the school and social problems his mood disorder had caused. After approximately one year of treatment, Napoleon was doing well in school with minimal behavioral issues.

CHRISTINA

Clinical History

Christina is a 12-year-old, black female who has been in foster care for the last two years because her mother died from HIV/AIDS. She resides with her foster parents (also her legal guardians) and two other foster children who are two and three years younger than she. At the strong encouragement of the Child Protective Services social worker, Christina was brought in for a psychiatric evaluation because she was sleeping *all* the time. Christina reluctantly admitted that she liked to sleep too much and did not like to talk about her emotions. When asked about her mother, she was very distant and aloof but admitted to missing her sometimes. Christina would not discuss the process of losing her mother or the disease that overcame her mother. In passing, the social worker reported that Christina was not doing as well in school lately and had been missing an excessive number of school days because she refused to get up for the bus. Christina denied ever seeing a therapist previously or taking any psychiatric medications.

Christina's mother contracted HIV from her father who was an intravenous heroin user. He died from HIV/AIDS during Christina's first year of life. Other psychiatric family history was basically unknown. According to the social worker, Christina has no other family involvement or support. Her developmental history was basically normal although her language was somewhat delayed.

Postcase Discussion and Diagnosis

Christina's symptoms have been further explored and revealed the following: experiencing depressed mood, feeling listless, feeling hopeless or helpless, having intermittent thoughts of wanting to die in order to join her mother, having poor appetite with a ten-pound-weight loss over the past month, feeling tired, having difficulty concentrating in school, and showing increased isolative behaviors. Christina was diagnosed with major depression, single episode, moderate (296.22) and needed immediate treatment. Given her thoughts of death, Christina needs to be carefully evaluated for suicidality. Psychotherapy is strongly recommended to address the enormous changes and losses that she has experienced in her short life. Although the issue of HIV transmission from mother to child should have already been addressed, the clinician needs to investigate and recommend an appropriate workup if necessary.

Proposed Psychopharmacological Treatment

Christina was started on fluoxetine (Prozac) 5 mg/d after consent was obtained from her foster parents. After two weeks, she was reevaluated and the fluoxetine was increased to 10 mg/d. After four weeks in treatment, she returned to the clinic with much less depression and isolation. She had also started psychotherapy to confront issues in her life. After taking the medication for ten weeks, Christina's depression had completely remitted and her therapy was progressing appropriately. She was beginning to process the loss of her mother and to look at how it had affected her own young life.

MARKY

Clinical History

Marky is an 8-year-old, white male who presented to the psychiatrist's office with both of his parents, although they are divorced. He was being brought in for evaluation at the recommendation of his third grade teacher, because he was disruptive in the classroom. His mother, who is the primary caretaker, reported he is always on the go and has trouble sitting still to do essentially anything. Marky's mother reported, "Everything in his room is in disarray." His father admitted that their son may be a little hyper but sees him as basically just a normal kid. The parents presented a letter from Marky's teacher that raised the following issues: difficulty attending to tasks, hyperactive in and out of the classroom, difficulty awaiting his turn, highly impulsive, difficulty following through with tasks, often procrastinates, frequently forgets, constantly daydreams, fights frequently, talks excessively, an so on. Marky has made average grades in school but has the potential to perform much better according to his teachers. Marky and his parents denied any significant depression, psychotic symptoms, obsessions, compulsions, or suicidality. Marky did admit to some anxiety and tends to worry mostly about the future.

Marky has always been in excellent health and tends to excel athletically. The parents denied any psychiatric family history of mental disorders or substance abuse. When giving the history, the father acknowledged that he also had trouble focusing in school when he was Marky's age. For this reason he tends to see Marky just as a normal child. Marky has never used any psychotropic medications in the past.

Postcase Discussion and Diagnosis

Marky clearly meets criteria for ADHD, combined type (314.01). After having the parents, teacher, and a family friend complete the Connors Rating Scale, the diagnosis was undisputed. The patient has features of hyperactivity, impulsivity, and inattention. The patient was also seen by his pediatrician who felt that Marky was healthy and developing normally.

Proposed Psychopharmacological Treatment

Marky and his parents agreed to a trial of Adderall XR (brand of amphetamine) starting at 5 mg every morning; the medication will be titrated up as tolerated every three to five days until Marky has a clinical response or has limiting side effects. A clinical response may be reported by the parents or child or objectively observed by a significant decrease in his Connors Rating Scale. The extended release (XR) form of the medication was chosen, because the medication is given as a single dose only in the morning, which helps improve compliance. Psychoeducation and therapy are necessary not only for the patient, but also for the family in order to ensure the best prognosis.

After being on Adderall XR 20 mg/d for a few days, Marky was functioning much better in school with improved self-confidence in his own abilities. His parents and teachers have noticed significant clinical improvements in his overall attitude, functioning, and demeanor. Marky had experienced no side effects to date from the psychostimulant. Objective measurements from the Connors Rating Scale showed Marky with lower scores that correlated with a therapeutic response.

CHAPTER SIXTEEN

CASE VIGNETTES: ADOLESCENTS

JOHNNY

Clinical History

Johnny is a 16-year-old, white male with no previous history of mental or physical illness. He recently presented to his family physician with complaints of depressed mood, loss of energy, poor motivation, and middle insomnia. His parents also mentioned that he had isolated from friends and dropped out of soccer. The history and physical showed no significant findings, but Johnny had lost seven pounds since his last physical about a year ago and appeared to be rather apathetic about personal hygiene. Johnny denied drug use, and while not presently suicidal, he did appear to have significant passive-death themes in this conversation.

Johnny's parents appeared to have a good relationship, and they appeared to have no concerns about Johnny's sister who is two years older than he. His sister had a brief period of depression last year, but it remitted without the need for further treatment. His mother, age 41, had several bouts of depression earlier in her life that resulted in a few years of psychotherapy and a course of antidepressant medication (imipramine) for several years. She claimed to have had no real depression over the last ten years. Johnny's father, age 45, reported that he occasionally is blue, but he had never felt the need to see a therapist or take medication. He does, however, drink two or more beers each evening when he gets home from work. He claimed that the beer calmed him and helped him sleep. Johnny's maternal grandfather committed suicide when Johnny's mother was three years old.

To date, Johnny has taken no medication and has only talked with the school counselor on three occasions about his depression and slumping grades. The counselor referred him back to his family physician for an assessment and gave him the name of a therapist in the area.

Postcase Discussion and Diagnosis

Johnny appears to have major depressive disorder (296.22). His score of 29 on the Beck Depression Inventory further confirms the presence of depression. He complains of poor motivation, death themes, tearful bouts, isolative behaviors, and trouble staying asleep at night. At this time, it is not certain if he will have subsequent bouts of depression, but based on the family's history, it is likely. While Johnny poses no immediate suicide risk, a timely evaluation by a mental-health professional is needed. Psychotherapy and medication are indicated. Johnny will see a local counselor at least twice a week for individual sessions and have an immediate medication and psychiatric evaluation with a psychiatrist.

Proposed Psychopharmacological Treatment

After the evaluation was completed, Johnny was placed on citalopram (Celexa) 10 mg/d for the first week and 20 mg/d starting in week two. This particular medication was selected because of its low overdose profile, low sedation, and its efficacy for facilitating sleep. Johnny will be watched closely by his parents and counselor for any changes in suicidal thoughts or behaviors. Follow-up sessions with the psychiatrist were scheduled in three-week intervals.

Upon follow-up with the counselor and the psychiatrist, Johnny reported that his depression was 80 percent better and that his grades had returned to normal. He no longer had trouble sleeping, nor was he plagued by thoughts of death and depression. He had decided to continue to talk with the counselor on an as needed basis since it helps him think more clearly and positively.

JENNIFER

Clinical History

Jennifer is a 17-year-old, Hispanic female who presented with anger, agitation, and antisocial tendencies. She lived with her parents until her father was sent to jail for an auto theft. Her mother who was unable to support herself and her three children on a farm worker's salary moved in with her sister and her five children. Jennifer had been in and out of school until she dropped out last year. She has about a sixth-grade-education achievement level. Her grades have always been poor, especially in reading and math. Jennifer claimed that she spent most of the fifth and sixth grades in the hall-way because of her poor behavior. She just cannot seem to listen and sit still long enough for things to stick. Her parents and teachers just thought of her as a headstrong tomboy who had to have the last word.

Jennifer's aunt had taken a strong interest in her behavior and believed that Jennifer should be able to have a decent educational experience. She had talked with Jennifer often and believed that she was "hyper and indifferent" to her current situation. Jennifer has spent much too much time with some neighborhood boys who have formed a type of gang with other young boys who have dropped out of the local high school. The neighborhood boys would rather skip school than attend and their grades were also poor. Jennifer's parents wanted to see her succeed in school but were more concerned that she would ruin her social reputation by hanging out with "bad boys."

They never really noticed her hyper behaviors before and just thought she had a lot of youthful energy. They feared she might become like many girls who hang with these boys and end up dropping out of school, getting into legal trouble, and getting pregnant before they are sixteen.

Reviews of Jennifer's past academic records showed poor performance and behavior patterns. She spent at least an hour a day in the hallway or in the principal's office when she last attended school last year. While Jennifer had little insight into her behavior, she was aware that school was not one of her favorite places and that she was not doing well there. She maintained that school was stupid and for geeks. Although she tended to hang with a rather antisocial crowd, she appeared to be concerned about her family and her other childhood friends. She appeared to have some sense of conscience, as she would not go with boys who planned vandalism or petty crimes. She was also very sensitive to other teens who had trouble learning in school and was often found talking with them in the cafeteria.

Postcase Discussion and Diagnosis

After extensive conversations with her former teachers, counselor, school psychologist, and social worker and a thorough workup from her family physician and her current psychologist, the team determined that Jennifer demonstrated enough clinical criteria for a diagnosis of ADHD of the hyperactive type. She was beginning to notice *less* hyperactivity and *more* restlessness with her life and her friends. Her self-esteem was rather low, because she realized that her educational skills were poor and her job prospects weak. With her psychologist's help, Jennifer was willing to work toward progress and improvement.

Proposed Psychopharmacologic Treatment

In addition to her weekly counseling sessions, Jennifer was sent to a psychiatrist who specializes in adult and childhood ADHD. She was initially started on a trial of atomoxetine (Strattera) but showed little response after one month. She was then switched to bupropion (Wellbutrin XL) 300 mg/d and methylphenidate (Ritalin) 15 mg bid. Her psychiatrist was not concerned about stimulant abuse, since Jennifer used no known substances. She responded well to this regime, as evidenced by self-reports and weekly reports from her psychologist. Subsequent psychological evaluations revealed that Jennifer had better concentration, attention, and retention of learned material.

In a series of follow-up sessions she demonstrated more calmness, less anger and agitation, and a willingness to enroll in a GED program. Her career and vocational tests indicated a strong interest and the ability to assist others in a counseling or teaching capacity. Jennifer hopes to become a teen counselor working with ADHD youth.

VIOLET

Clinical History

Violet is a 15-year-old female in the ninth grade. She came with her parents to a local mental health center complaining of intense anxiety and social shyness. The visit was prompted by a rather traumatic school dance; Violet came home early with her friend, Lisa, at Violet's insistence. Violet reported that she was feeling more and more uncomfortable at the dance, and when she mentioned her feelings to Lisa, her friend told her "lighten up" and stop obsessing about everything. Violet became quite upset and started to cry. Others at the dance gathered around her until school personnel escorted Violet and Lisa from the building. Violet's parents were called and the two girls were taken home.

Violet is the older of two children. She has an 11-year-old brother who has no apparent mental health concerns. Her parents appeared to be happy and well adjusted with no history of mental illness, however, her mother reported that she was rather anxious herself in high school and college. Violet's mother took nortriptyline (Pamelor) for several years, but reported no anxiety problems now.

Both parents claimed that Violet had always been a shy, quiet, and very sensitive little girl. She was always uncomfortable around strangers and other students. In fact, she had a difficult time adjusting to both kindergarten and first grade. Although she is a very pretty girl, Violet avoided social contact with other students, and quickly excused herself when approached by them. Recently, while Violet was visiting at Lisa's home, a few more friends showed up and suggested calling some boys over. Violet became more and more anxious until she excused herself and retreated to Lisa's bedroom. Lisa called Violet's mom who came to take her home.

Violet is aware that her fears and behaviors are ruining her life. She reported that she felt very inadequate in social situations. Violet is afraid that she will do or say something that will bring attention to her, and others will laugh at her. She also reported feeling very uncomfortable in the girl's shower room at school. Violet will not shower or dress unless the other students have gone. She once became so concerned that others were watching her that she had trouble breathing and felt dizzy.

After a complete physical by her family doctor and an evaluation by the therapist in the clinic, no physical causes for Violet's anxiety were found. She functioned quite well at home and in the presence of people she knew well. School performance was good except when she had to raise her hand or give speeches in front of the class. She appeared to have no other phobias, history of depression, and no history of trauma or abuse.

Postcase Discussion and Diagnosis

Violet appears to have social phobia (300.23). She has always been rather shy and anxious in social situations, but recently her symptoms have worsened. She purposely avoids social situations and the possibilities of social invitations. She once dropped a class because the teacher said the students would have to work in groups. She fears that if her anxieties continue, she will not be able to finish high school or attend college.

Proposed Psychopharmacological Treatment

In addition to cognitive-behavioral therapy and social-skills training classes, her therapist and parents decided that Violet should try medication. She was first given paroxetine (Paxil) 20 mg/day. She responded very well but reported feeling rather drugged during the day. Her yawning was so pronounced that her teachers excused her from class to sleep in the student lounge. She was then instructed to take the medication before bed, which helped, but sedation and dizziness continued to be a problem. She was then switched to venlafaxine (Effexor XR) and showed less sedation and balance issues.

A follow-up found that Violet was much happier and certainly more social. Once the medication reduced her fears, Violet opened up to the therapist and really worked hard on finding ways to reduce her fears and increase her strengths. The social skills classes increased her self-esteem and allowed her to address her fear that everyone must like her.

In a true *in-vivo* test, she attended a school dance recently and actually accepted a boy's invitation to dance. She was quite smitten with him and is now wearing his school ring.

CHAPTER SEVENTEEN

CASE VIGNETTES: EARLY ADULTHOOD

STONE

Clinical History

Stone is a 23-year-old, white male, college student who presented to the Campus Health Center with concerns about failing health. Upon further questioning, the patient reported concerns about microwaves, X rays, and other electromagnetic forces interfering with his decision-making capacity. Although he was initially guarded, Stone confided that he stopped watching television one year ago and stopped listening to the radio six months ago because he felt like "the government" was trying to control his mind. At times, the patient referred to hearing his "mother and father" in his head but refused to elaborate when questioned.

Stone had been attending college for the past four years and had approximately one more year to finish his bachelor's degree in chemistry. Stone remorsefully admitted to drinking and smoking "too much weed" that led to his withdrawal from about half of his classes during his first and second years of college. Stone denied any current use of drugs, but he did admit to having some alcohol about once a month with friends. Further assessment of his alcohol history revealed two positive answers out of a possible four on the CAGE questionnaire. Stone reported that he did not date much and preferred to be alone. He casually mentioned having some friends but was reluctant to give any names or reveal anything specific. Despite his initial complaint of failing health, his review of systems was basically negative.

Stone denied any significant medical history except for surgery on a broken arm when he was about 15 years old. When questioned about psychiatric family history, Stone admitted that his maternal grandfather had a "nervous breakdown" and was institutionalized most of his adult life. Stone admitted that his grandfather used to hallucinate and "act weird," he was unsure of the diagnosis. Stone reported that his father drinks too much alcohol and has had one DUI in the past. Stone denied any particular stressors lately except for the pressure he was getting from his parents to finish college and get a job.

Postcase Discussion and Diagnosis

According to Stone's history, he appears to have a diagnosis of schizophrenia, paranoid type (295.30), alcohol abuse (305.00), and cannabis abuse (305.20). Additional information about Stone revealed few relationships, increasing isolation over the last few years, increasing paranoid delusions, and intermittent auditory hallucinations. His school performance was average but appeared to be declining overall when compared to his high school years. He was ambivalent about discussing his concerns with others because he feared his health would deteriorate. Stone's use of alcohol and marijuana complicated his presentation but was probably an independent phenomenon. If his substance abuse continues or progresses, his psychotic disorder will likely worsen. Stone's family history most likely indicated his maternal grandfather had either schizophrenia or some other psychotic illness. Although Stone desired to process his thoughts and feelings in therapy, he was not an appropriate candidate given his subacute psychotic symptoms. At some later point in time, therapy may be appropriate. Before considering medication, Stone was referred for an appropriate medical and neurological examination

Proposed Psychopharmacological Treatment

Stone was started on aripiprazole (Abilify) 10 mg/d because he felt safe taking a neuromodulator, rather than some of the other atypical neuroleptics. Given his chemistry background, he was suspicious of being prescribed anything he felt was a tranquilizer. After four weeks on the medication, Stone reported very little change in his symptomatology. He appeared to be tolerating the medication well without any side effects. At eight weeks, Stone appeared much more relaxed and focused on completing school rather than being obsessed with his "failing health." When asked about his health at this point, Stone denied having any problems and was even listening to the radio in his car again. Furthermore, at twelve weeks of aripiprazole 10 mg/d, he reported having a potential girlfriend in his chemistry class. Since his psychosis was responding to the medication, psychotherapy should be initiated with the focus on psychoeducation, relapse prevention, and avoidance of substances.

AVA

Clinical History

Ava is a 27-year-old, Hispanic-Asian homemaker and mother of a 3-year-old daughter. She was accompanied to the clinic by her husband of six years with a complaint of unusual behaviors. Ava had been taking walks in the middle of the night when she was unable to sleep, had become fearful of her husband for no apparent reason, and was consuming and hiding alcohol at various places in their home. Her husband reported that Ava did not usually drink alcohol whatsoever because of their religious beliefs. Upon further questioning, Ava revealed that she was six weeks pregnant and the father of the baby was not her husband. Both Ava and her husband were unwilling to reveal much information about the pregnancy except to say that they would remain married and raise the child as their own.

When asked about historical information, Ava said that she had a "strange episode" about seven years earlier when she impulsively took a vacation with a college friend. After drinking excessively for one month, Ava returned to school to learn that she had failed her semester classes. She did not seek any mental health treatment and thought her behavior was just related to "growing up."

With the exception of alcohol, Ava had no history of other drug use. She had never taken any previous psychiatric medications. The psychiatric family history was negative for mood disorders, psychotic disorders, anxiety disorders, and substance-use disorders. During the interview, Ava acknowledged other symptoms, including increased energy, moodiness (dysphoria, elation, and irritability), racing thoughts, hearing the voice of God, feeling like she is "God's chosen one," and cleaning excessively at home.

Ava saw her primary care physician who felt she was in good health. The physician advised her not to drink alcohol while she is pregnant because of fetal-alcohol concerns and referred her for follow up with her OB/GYN. Ava currently takes a prenatal vitamin only.

Postcase Discussion and Diagnosis

Ava appears to have a diagnosis of bipolar disorder, manic, severe with psychotic features (296.34) and alcohol abuse (305.00). Her symptoms that support this diagnosis include hyperreligiosity, grandiose delusions, mild paranoia, racing thoughts, decreased need for sleep, increased goal-directed activities, auditory hallucinations, impulsivity, possible hypersexuality, and poor judgment. Her intermittent alcohol consumption may be a form of self-medication to control her mania. Based on Ava's history, she probably had at least one manic episode previously that went undiagnosed and untreated. In addition to referring Ava for medication evaluation and treatment, the clinician needs to provide psychotherapeutic support to her and her husband and ensure the safety of her daughter. Ava's husband agreed to enlist support of relatives to provide childcare and support for Ava until she gets back to her old self.

Proposed Psychopharmacological Treatment

After an appropriate evaluation and review of all options available, Ava and her husband chose to start lithium 300 mg bid initially, with dosage adjustments over the next few weeks. Because of her psychosis, antipsychotics were discussed, but Ava and her husband decided to wait for now and see how she responds to the lithium. After two weeks of lithium, Ava was sleeping about seven hours per night, had less racing thoughts, and was abstinent from alcohol. Her husband reported a significant improvement from his perspective saying, "my wife is coming back." The lithium was increased to 300 mg tid at that time; the lithium level subsequently was 0.8 mEq/l, which was therapeutic. In consultation with her OB/GYN, an ultrasound was done to check for cardiac abnormalities in the fetus because of the lithium exposure. Results were negative indicating that the fetus was unaffected. Given Ava's alcohol abuse, the possibility of fetal-alcohol effects needs to be assessed after delivery.

CANDY

Clinical History:

Candy is a 25-year-old, white female who presented for an evaluation at the insistence of her primary care physician because of weight loss. Candy reported that she felt overweight, fat, and disgusted with her appearance. She claimed, "My thighs, stomach, and butt are just too fat. . . . I have to lose more weight." Candy acknowledged some depression but tended to minimize it, saying she was fine. She denied any sleep disturbance, energy changes, hopelessness, helplessness, concentration problems, suicidality, and so on. She reported having a normal appetite but was very careful to eat only "healthy foods." When asked about stressors, she admitted to some trouble in her marriage but did not elaborate. Candy works as an attorney. She reported that she gets angry at clients and even judges when "things" don't go her way. She exercises daily for approximately one hour, focusing on aerobics and cardiovascular fitness. Her stats are as follows: height, 5'8," weight, 98 pounds; and BMI 14.9 kg/m^2. According to standard measurements, her BMI is in the 2nd percentile. She mentioned in passing that her doctor was concerned because she has not had a menstrual period for the last two years.

Candy went on to report that she had been obsessed with her weight since her teenage years. She remembered constantly struggling with her parents over control issues such as clothing, school performance, friends, dating, and so on. She denied any significant past medical or psychiatric history, as well as any alcohol or drug abuse. Her psychiatric family history revealed some depression in her mother and maternal grandmother. Candy also stated, "Nobody in my family is fat and I'm not going to be either." In passing, she reluctantly admitted to sexual abuse in the past but refused to discuss details.

Postcase Discussion and Diagnosis

Candy presents with a diagnosis of anorexia nervosa (307.1) and may have a secondary diagnosis of depressive disorder. She is excessively focused on body image and has an intense fear of gaining weight despite being underweight. She appears to be in the acute phase of the illness although she has not experienced any medical consequences to date other than her amenorrhea. It is difficult to assess whether Candy has experienced depressive episodes in the past because of her vague history. She does not meet criteria for a specific diagnosis of mood or anxiety disorder at this time. Candy does need appropriate laboratory evaluation to check for electrolyte abnormalities, which could be medically dangerous. An appropriate trial of psychotherapy should be initiated as well as evaluating her need for inpatient hospitalization.

Proposed Psychopharmacological Treatment

Although most data would not suggest treating the acute phase with medications, Candy agreed to a trial of fluoxetine (Prozac) 10 mg/d for one week, then 20 mg/d. She understood that the medication may help her mood as well as decrease her core eating disorder symptoms. The fluoxetine was increased over the next four weeks to 60 mg/d, which she tolerated well without side effects. After approximately six weeks on the fluoxetine, Candy appeared to be less depressed and less obsessed with her weight. Over the subsequent six weeks, her weight increased to 104 pounds and she appeared to be unconcerned about it. The combination of psychotherapy and medication management has provided Candy with the best possible prognosis. Ongoing psychotherapy, medications, and psychoeducation will be required to maintain her emotional health chronically.

CHAPTER EIGHTEEN

CASE VIGNETTES: MIDDLE ADULTHOOD

CHESTER

Clinical History

Chester is a 42-year-old, white male seeking an evaluation at a university-based treatment center. He decided to consult the experts, because he had tried so many other treatments in the past with mixed results. He presented with a history of panic attacks dating back to high school. His first attack came during his senior year when he was not accepted to Princeton. This rejection was a terrible blow to his self-esteem, because his father attended Princeton and expected that both Chester and his brother would also attend. His brother was then in his junior year and planning to attend law school when finished.

After Chester's first attack in high school, he and his parents consulted their doctor and a cardiologist who found no reason for the attacks and no heart-related issues. Chester was told to reduce his stress and return if the attacks continued. They did not return and Chester was accepted to Harvard, an acceptable alternative. In his freshman year, Chester experienced another attack while he was sleeping. He consulted the university health services, which once again found no medical reason for the attacks, and they explained to him that the attacks may be a stress-related condition. An appointment was made for him at the university counseling service, but he did not show for the appointment.

Chester made it through college by using alcohol to self-medicate. He was able to hide most of his drinking from his family and friends until he graduated and met Judy. He and Judy fell in love and married within six months. His drinking became harder to hide, and Judy confronted him after he fell at a neighbor's party where he was very drunk and rather loud. Chester confided in her about his panic and fears, and how he needs the alcohol to function at home and at work. With Judy's help, he decided to attend AA and seek counseling from a mental health professional.

Chester slowly refrained from drinking but felt increasingly more anxious until he had three panic attacks in one week. He was placed on alprazolam (Xanax) by a consulting psychiatrist. He found the medication very helpful and was able to learn how to identify, label, and modify his thoughts in counseling with the use of cognitive therapy. He attended therapy weekly for nearly two years, but stopped when he and the therapist felt they had progressed far enough. He continued to take the medication and remained symptom free for over fourteen years.

When he was 36 years old, his primary care physician believed that Chester was over his emotional concerns. His physician felt Chester should stop taking the alprazolam. Over the years, Chester had increased his dose from 0.5 mg/day to over 3 mg/day. He still attended AA meetings from time to time but never touched alcohol again. By the second week of his step down from alprazolam, Chester experienced a panic attack while driving home from work. His medication was increased back to 3 mg/day of alprazolam and has remained at this dose for the past six years. He attempted to return to therapy, but found the principles of therapy were not helping him much this time around. Chester changed therapists, but the next therapist was less versed than the first, adding to his sense of failure.

About a month ago Chester's 17-year-old son was accepted to Princeton. Although happy for his son, Chester became very depressed and while shopping with his wife in a grocery store, he experienced an intense panic attack. He is tired of partially effective approaches and desires a more comprehensive form of treatment.

Postcase Discussion and Diagnosis

Chester has a long history of panic disorder without agoraphobia (300.01), with secondary, alcohol and sedative-hypnotic abuse. While he used alcohol to self-medicate early in his life, he abused the benzodiazepine alprazolam later in his life. Both drugs offered some level of immediate relief but did not provide a permanent solution to his concerns.

Proposed Psychopharmacologic Treatment

Since Chester has such a long and chronic history of panic disorder, it is very likely that he will continue to experience panic, especially if he attempts to reduce his dose of alprazolam. Since cognitively based psychotherapy helped him before, he should try it again. The use of antidepressants, especially SSRIs, are very helpful in reducing or eliminating panic. Chester will be placed on an SSRI such as fluoxetine (Prozac), sertraline (Zoloft), or citalopram (Celexa), and he will be reevaluated every two weeks to determine drug effectiveness. Concurrently, the alprazolam will be very slowly tapered off in increments of 0.25 mg/week. Good patient education will be needed to help Chester understand that he will not have additional panic attacks once the antidepressant medication takes effect.

In a five month follow-up, Chester was symptom free and attending counseling twice per month. He continues to take the SSRI but no longer uses benzodiazepines or alcohol for symptom relief. He also attends a group for others with panic disorder called Agoraphobics in Motion.

SALLY

Clinical History

Sally is a 47-year-old, white female who was married for nearly twenty years when her husband Jack asked her for a divorce. While she loved Jack, she admitted that they had fallen out of love many years ago. They had a very civil divorce when their only daughter Amy was a senior in high school. Amy appeared to be the only person in the home who was upset about the divorce, and Sally was there to be supportive. Amy is now in her junior year at a university more than 1500 miles away. While Amy comes home for major holidays, she spends little time with Sally or with her father who lives in an apartment in a nearby town. While this tends to upset Sally more than Jack, Sally is trying to understand that college kids would rather spend more time with their old high school friends than with their parents.

After the divorce, Sally started to spend more time with her own parents. They were well into their seventies. While she loved her father, she was closer to her mother. Sally too was an only child, and she often stopped by her parent's home just to check in on them. One Sunday morning Sally received a call from her mother; her father had a heart attack. He was pronounced dead before he arrived at the emergency room. Sally and her mother were devastated, but Sally tried to be strong for her mother. Her mother moved in with Sally and Sally started to care for her. Sally started spending less and less time with others. She never went out with friends or coworkers, in fact, the only time Sally left the house was to go to work or take her mother on errands.

Sally began to notice that she was isolating more and was growing more depressed. Her sleep was problematic since her father died and it was not getting better. Sally tried to treat the initial insomnia with over-the-counter sleep aids, but they offered only temporary assistance. She would also experience terminal insomnia two to three times per week. Sally was also growing more concerned that she seldom saw or heard from her daughter. She once took a trip to see Amy at the university, but Amy was away on an extended field trip.

When Sally returned from her trip to see Amy, she found that her mother had a very serious cold. When her mother's breathing became labored, Sally took her to a local urgent-care center and her mother was immediately hospitalized with pneumonia. Her condition continued to decline until she was placed on a respirator. Four days later Sally's mother died. Sally was overwhelmed with grief. She phoned her daughter who came home but only stayed until the day of the funeral. Amy claimed that she needed to return to school to prepare for her LSAT exam.

Sally was tearful nearly twenty-four hours a day. She barely slept, and the sleep remedies offered no relief. She attempted to see her minister, but he referred her to a grief group. She attended meetings for several weeks but found that the grief of others made her worse. Sally attempted to return to work but could not concentrate or do her job well. After more than six months, her grief and loss was still very much with her. She felt that she may need to consult a mental health professional for the first time in her life.

Postcase Discussion and Diagnosis

While Sally clearly exhibited all clinical criteria for a major depressive episode, which should be considered in her treatment approach, she most certainly demonstrated a complicated bereavement. Sally often dreamed of her mother, and once she thought that she heard her mother calling out to her and asking for assistance because she had fallen down the basement steps. Sally raced down the stairs in the middle of the night only to find that her cat was locked outside and wanted in for the night. Sally feels she cannot continue to live in the house, because it has too many reminders of her mother around. She has basically sealed off the guest room where her mother slept and is afraid to touch her things.

When Sally's father died, she did not have an opportunity to grieve. She had to be strong for her mother and daughter. Sally wanted to be comforted but could not find this in her own daughter. Sally had few close friends to confide in, but her bond with her mother was close. When her mother died, the only bond Sally ever really had was broken and lost. She realized that the bond with Amy was weak and unreliable. Sally panicked thinking about her own vulnerabilities. Who would care for her when she got sick? Who would grieve for her? Did she fail as a mother? Why did her daughter distance herself?

Proposed Psychopharmacologic Treatment

Sally was evaluated at a comprehensive health and mental care facility. After a complete physical, change-of-life issues where assessed by her gynecologist. Her gynecologist suggested appropriate hormone replacement and referred Sally to a counselor who specialized in grief therapy. Since Sally's depressive symptoms have been severe for so long, she was referred to a physician for medication. She was placed on Wellbutrin XL, 150 mg/d (brand of bupropion). While this medication did offer some relief from depression, Sally reported feeling rather agitated during the day and her sleep disturbances continued. She was switched to sertraline (Zoloft), which improved her sleep but increased her irritable bowel symptoms. Finally, Sally was placed on trazodone (Desyrel), which offered the antidepressant action with sedation around the time for sleep.

Upon follow-up three months later, Sally reported feeling much less depressed. Her sleep had returned to normal without disturbing dreams. She felt that she was able to "move on" now and let mother rest. She continues to take the medication and see the counselor when needed. Sally approached her daughter on her last trip home. Her daughter did not realize just how far that they had drifted apart, and Sally vowed to try harder to bridge the gap between them.

TONY

Clinical History

Tony is a 50-year-old, Asian male with a long history of severe depression. He is the oldest of three siblings who were raised in the suburbs of Philadelphia. His parents owned a dry cleaning and tailoring business; each family member worked there as well. Tony's family were devout Catholics and expected each child to attend a Catholic school. Tony's parents hoped that he would get a scholarship to Notre Dame or Georgetown University. Tony was a good student and did in fact earn a scholarship to Georgetown.

Tony first noticed his depression at age fourteen. He was afraid that he was different from other boys, because he found other boys attractive. He never mentioned his fear to his parents, because the family never really talked about problems in the home. Tony did not want to disrespect his family by talking to an outsider about his concerns, so he kept it to himself. During his years at Georgetown, the depression became quite severe, and Tony had to inform his family about it. As often seen in Asian families, they were disappointed in him for having a mental illness. Tony never told them he was gay.

At the insistence of a professor, Tony entered therapy and started taking nortriptyline for his depression. He showed enough improvement to finish his degree and move to Detroit to start a new job in engineering. Tony functioned fairly well for about six years until he decided to stop the medication due to weight gain and other side effects. He experienced a serious depressive episode that led to a fairly lengthy hospitalization. Tony was reintroduced to nortriptyline, but this time it would not work. He was finally placed on trazodone (Desyrel) and clonazepam (Klonopin) because of his agitation and related anxiety. When he was released, he attended day hospital for several weeks. Although Tony was functioning fairly well, he believed that he was only 65 percent better.

The next eight years demonstrated Tony's need for additional medications and increases in medications already in use. He was introduced to various SSRIs as they arrived on the treatment scene, but each offered only moderate effectiveness. Numerous consultations with experts at both Wayne State University and the University of Michigan lead to various polypharmacologic approaches. Tony demonstrated only moderated levels of improvement to lithium augmentation and stimulant boosters. He refused to try MAOIs because of their dietary restrictions.

Tony was able to return to work, but he took so much sick time that he was transferred to a less-stressful department. The transfer resulted in a pay cut that Tony viewed as a demotion.

After years of psychotherapy, Tony finally felt comfortable with his sexual orientation and decided to tell his family. While his sisters were supportive, his parents were not. They never missed an opportunity to tell him about "change therapies" and the "evils" of a gay lifestyle. Tony stopped returning to Philadelphia to see them. Over time, the rejections had somewhat of a "kindling effect," that is, these stressors were setting off subsequent bouts of depression that were becoming more severe.

Feeling more comfortable with his gay identity, Tony was able to venture out a bit and meet others. He met another man, and they started to date. This man was very understanding about Tony's chronic depression and tried to help Tony with some of his issues. Since this friend had a very accepting family, Tony quickly felt welcomed and accepted by them, but he continued to obsess over the loss of his own family.

Over the next few years, Tony and his partner, Bob, set up housekeeping, but Tony's numerous hospitalizations and leaves from work led him to apply for permanent disability. Tony was granted disability, but unfortunately he spent his time lying around the house sleeping. He isolated and refused to speak to anyone other than Bob. Except for his sisters, Tony had no contact with his family, who viewed his gayness and his mental illness as a major stigma (not unusual in an Asian family). Both Tony and Bob felt there must be more-effective forms of treatment.

Postcase Discussion and Diagnosis

Tony is suffering from major depression with a rather chronic history (296.32). While he has never been actively suicidal, his chronic depressive episodes have left him feeling that life is not worth living. He does not abuse alcohol or other drugs, and there are no psychotic manifestations to his illness. While his homosexuality was rather ego dystonic at first, Tony appears to have made a healthy adjustment to it in the last few years. The family stressors continue, but Tony is happy with the relationship he has with his sisters and Bob's family.

Proposed Psychopharmacologic Treatment

Tony had been tried on every known TCA, SSRI, and heterocyclic. Various stimulant and lithium boosters were not very helpful. A recent augmentation with olanzepine (Zyprexa) showed little change. Even though Tony was opposed to the use of MAOIs, their use was reevaluated with him. With his psychologist's help, Tony was educated about possible MAOI use and informed of the possible benefits. He reluctantly agreed to try them, and after the appropriate discontinuance period from the other medications, he was started on phenelzine (Nardil), 30 mg/d. Initially his depression worsened after the discontinuance of the other medications, but by the third week on phenelzine, Tony was beginning to improve. His dose was increased to 60 mg/d, and by the sixth week of treatment, he was reporting less daytime sleeping, no tearful bouts, and a much improved affect. Bob reported that Tony was helping him in the yard, asking to see their friends, and joining him for family visits.

The final evaluation came three months after the phenelzine was started. Tony reported no measurable depression. He is not working as an engineer, but he is working three half-days per week in a bookstore and loves his job. He reported that he and Bob are getting along well. Tony is planning a trip home at Christmas to see his parents; he believes that he is ready to see them and to confront their issues with his depression and sexual identity.

CHAPTER NINETEEN

CASE VIGNETTES: OLDER ADULTHOOD

ROSE

Clinical History

Rose is an 82-year-old, white female who presented for a psychiatric evaluation with a referral from her primary care physician. According to Rose, "My doctor was concerned about my memory, but I think it is fine." Rose lives alone in a mobile home with her two cats. She reported that she had no family to help her, because they are all deceased. Rose was accompanied to the appointment by a long-time friend who drives her to the store and other appointments. Rose admitted to feeling sad but denied feeling depressed on a consistent basis. She worried about the future now that she was getting old, but knew that she would be taken care of one way or another. She stated, "My memory is not as good as it used to be, but I get by okay." She does not drink anymore but used to enjoy an occasional martini with friends. Rose reported some difficulty sleeping but denied any energy disturbance, appetite disturbance, difficulty concentrating, hopeless feelings, helpless feelings, or thoughts of death.

According to her friend, Rose is having significant difficulty with her memory. For example, twice within the past two weeks she had forgotten to turn off the stove after preparing a meal. Rose frequently lost her mail, bills, and social security checks, but generally they were just misplaced. In the past six months, Rose's electricity had been shut off once and her water had been shut off twice because of nonpayment. When asked about her finances, Rose reported that everything is fine. She was unable to provide further details even when directly asked. Her friend stated that Rose was forgetting to feed her animals and at times she even forgot to eat. Information from Rose's primary care physician revealed an 18-month history of cognitive decline as well as various medical diagnoses including hypertension, osteoarthritis, and a previous history of myocardial infarction. She is currently taking an antihypertensive medication as well as an arthritis medication, which has remained unchanged for the last seven years. Her primary care physician also noted that Rose was more forgetful, called him by the wrong name at times, and no longer knew the names of her medications.

While her mental status was essentially unremarkable, Rose tended to avoid current events and did not know the names of the president or vice president. She tended to minimize her deficits saying, ". . . they're no good anyway."

Postcase Discussion and Diagnosis

Rose appears to have dementia of the Alzheimer's type (294.10). Her mini-mental status exam (MMSE) is 15/30 (-5 orientation, -2 attention, -2 recall, -2 naming, -2 command, -1 writing sentence, -1 copy). Rose has additional symptoms including aphasia, apraxia, agnosia, and problems with executive functioning. She has also been evaluated recently by a neurologist who ordered an MRI of the brain that showed moderate atrophy. The neurologist agreed with the dementia diagnosis and did not feel any further workup was necessary. In addition, Rose who was quite distressed at hearing the diagnosis needed a referral for psychotherapy to address these issues. Her primary care physician indicated that Rose uses atenolol, 50 mg/day for her hypertension and Tylenol, 2 pills/day (over the counter) for her arthritis.

Proposed Psychopharmacological Treatment

Rose was started on donepezil (Aricept), 5 mg/d for the first four weeks, then 10 mg/d thereafter. She appeared to tolerate the medication well except for mild sedation. When the dosing was changed from the morning to the evening, the sedation side effect resolved. Her medications were reviewed and no significant drug interactions between the atenolol, Tylenol, and donepezil were found. Rose was able to continue living in her current environment, but four hours daily of home-care assistance were added. This care will help ensure compliance with her medication, adequacy of meals, cleanliness of her home, and so on. Rose allowed her long-time friend and her accountant to take over her finances and pay the monthly expenses.

Rose initially attended psychotherapy sessions weekly, but sessions were tapered to monthly by the end of six months. The individual psychotherapy appeared to help Rose adjust to the enormous changes that were occurring in her life. After six months of treatment with donepezil, her MMSE was 14/30. Following one year of treatment, Rose was still living at home, had eight hours of home care daily, and had a MMSE of 15/30. Since she is still living independently with the same basic MMSE score, the medication to minimize her cognitive decline has definitely been efficacious.

ANTHONY

Clinical History

Anthony is a 65-year-old, black male who presented for psychiatric evaluation with his daughter. Anthony revealed that he lost his wife suddenly fifteen months ago after a fatal myocardial infarction. He reported, "We were married for forty years. . . . I don't know what to do now." His daughter reported that nothing had been the same since her mother died. She further mentioned, "My dad has been isolating himself to the point of being a recluse." The patient admited that the isolation was true along with other symptoms including early and middle insomnia, decreased appetite with a 25-pound-weight loss over the past year, decreased energy, poor concentration, and increased forgetfulness. When questioned about suicide, Anthony reported thoughts of wanting to join his wife, but he had no acute suicide plan or intent. He drank one glass of red wine daily for the last twenty years without any history of abuse. Because he and his wife used to do almost everything together, Anthony was feeling very lonely and had much survivor's guilt.

Anthony, whose only medication is one aspirin and a multivitamin daily, had been evaluated by his internist and given a good bill of health. He denied any personal history of depression or emotional problems or any in his family. He reported that his daughter and extended family were supportive, but life was just not the same without his wife. Anthony had used spiritual resources that had been somewhat helpful at times, but he seemed to fall back again into the mourning process.

In addition, Anthony reported increasing forgetfulness and memory dysfunction over the past year. There was no pattern or consistency to his cognitive dysfunction. According to him, "Some days I can remember recent things . . . some days I can remember past things." Furthermore, his daughter reported that he had stopped his morning walks and had dropped out of his bowling league.

Postcase Discussion and Diagnosis

Anthony clearly has the diagnosis of major depression, single episode, moderate (296.22). Upon further interview, the patient had significantly worsened over the past three months, which was the first anniversary of his wife's death. His depressive episode has been further characterized by anhedonia, isolation, distractibility, hopelessness, helplessness, and worthlessness. In order to evaluate the memory complaints, a MMSE was completed during his initial visit with the score being 27/30 (-1 orientation, -1 attention, -1 recall). His effort on this examination was poor due to his level of depression. He was referred for psychotherapy to help facilitate the grieving process, which was most likely the root of his clinical depression.

Proposed Psychopharmacological Treatment

Anthony was started on sertraline (Zoloft), 25 mg/d for week one, then 50 mg/d thereafter. He had requested this medication after seeing an advertisement on TV. After taking the medication for two weeks, it was unclear whether he was benefiting or not. He reported having no side effects. At that time, the sertraline was increased to 75 mg/d for the third week, then 100 mg/d thereafter. During his next visit, he reported a moderate response to the sertraline 100 mg/d after taking it for two weeks. The only side effect he reported was mild loosening of his bowel movements, which was tolerable. Anthony engaged in psychotherapy with full remission of his grief and depression and even invited his daughter to a few sessions. At three months in treatment, his

MMSE was 30/30 revealing that he was cognitively intact. The initial cognitive dysfunction was due to his depression rather than to a dementing process. Again, the combination of psychotherapy and medication management was helpful in restoring Anthony's previous level of functioning.

MARGARITA

Clinical History

Margarita is a 70-year-old, Hispanic-American female who was referred by her primary care physician and managed-care plan for ongoing evaluation and treatment. She stated her chief complaint insisting, "I need my medication doctor . . . I can't go without it or I'll get sick again." The patient gave a long psychiatric history with multiple psychiatric hospitalizations dating back to her twenties. She now reported that a man was bothering her, making sexual advances to her, and frequently attempting to have "brain sex" with her. Upon further questioning, she reported hearing his voice at night through the walls in her single-family home. She got rather upset, angry, and paranoid that this was happening to her and frequently called the police for help. She stated, "The police don't even try to help me anymore . . .. they say that he is not real." Margarita went on to report "strange sensations" on her skin when she was out in public (e.g., grocery store or bank) and related these sensations to men looking at her amorously. She has siblings and other relatives but refuses contact with them saying they are "cursed." The patient also reported a history of depression and moodiness with one previous suicide attempt by overdosing about fifteen years ago.

Margarita is currently taking chlorpromazine (Thorazine), 500 mg/d, diazepam (Valium), 30 mg/d, imipramine (Tofranil), 100 mg/d, and chloral hydrate (Notec) 500 mg/d. She also takes antihypertensive medication, an oral agent for her diabetes, and an inhaler for her emphysema. She reported that she had been on this psychiatric medication regimen for years with marginal functioning. She had a history of alcohol abuse when she was in her thirties and forties and reported that the alcohol helped decrease her mood swings. Her psychiatric family history revealed that her paternal grandmother was institutionalized in a sanitarium, and her maternal aunt had depression with multiple suicide attempts. The family had no history of substance abuse. Margarita's social history revealed that she was different from her peers even in her teens. She attempted college but dropped out because she could not concentrate and focus on her work. Although she had never been employed, she had been financially supported by a trust fund from her father who was a wealthy businessman in Mexico.

Postcase Discussion and Diagnosis

Margarita has the diagnosis of schizoaffective disorder, bipolar type (295.70). Observation of her during the interview revealed mild-moderate tardive dyskinesia of the face and upper extremities resulting from years of exposure to the typical neuroleptics. She appeared very isolated and lonely, but had most likely created this scenario given her chronic psychiatric disability. Although Margarita never had a clear manic episode, she had experienced mixed-mood states that were indicative of the bipolar type of the diagnosis. Medication changes could be extremely helpful in decreasing her psychotic mood symptoms.

Proposed Psychopharmacological Treatment

After developing some trust with the patient over a few weeks time, her psychiatrist adjusted her medications to an alternative regimen that should be more helpful. The chlorpromazine 500 mg/d was replaced gradually by risperidone (Risperdal) 3–4 mg/d for her psychotic symptoms, which seemed to be the most bothersome at this time. Subsequently, the diazepam and chloral hydrate were tapered slowly over a period of six to eight weeks. Topiramate (Topamax) was a logical alternative to replace these two medications given Margarita's mood instability, insomnia, and anxiety. After these changes were implemented, the imipramine was reevaluated and tapered to reduce her polypharmacy regimen. She should not be given benzodiazepines because of her history of alcohol abuse.

After six months of treatment, Margarita was taking risperidone 3 mg/d and topiramate 200 mg/d without any significant side effects. She still had some unusual thoughts and concerns, but she was functioning much better on a daily basis with an improved quality of life. The tardive dyskinesia was still present at the same level, but it will not be progressive with this atypical antipsychotic drug regimen.

APPENDIX

TABLE OF PSYCHOTROPIC MEDICATIONS

Abbreviations used in the table include the following:

DA (dopamine), EPS (extra pyramidal symptoms),
GABA (gamma-aminobutyric acid), H (histamine),
5 HT (serotonin), M (muscarinic), NE (norepinephrine),
NMS (neuroleptic malignant syndrome),
WBC (white blood count)

GENERIC NAME (DRUG CLASS)	TRADE/BRAND NAME	MECHANISM OF ACTION	TYPICAL DOSE (MG/DAY)	MOST COMMON SIDE EFFECTS
acamprosate (antialcohol)	Campral	GABA receptor modifier	2000–3000	Diarrhea, dyspepsia, headache, nausea, vomiting, rash
alprazolam (antianxiety)	Xanax, Xanax XR	Increases GABA	0.25–4	Poor coordination, dizziness, sedation, weakness, memory dysfunction, depression, lethargy
amantadine (antiparkinsonian)	Symmetrel	DA agonist	100–300	Nausea, dizziness, insomnia, dry mouth, constipation, confusion, fatigue, anxiety
amitriptyline (antidepressant)	Elavil	5-HT reuptake inhibition, NE reuptake inhibition	150–300	Sedation, weight gain, dry mouth, blurry vision, constipation, urinary retention, sexual dysfunction, orthostatic hypotension, dizziness
amoxapine (antidepressant)	Ascendin	NE reuptake inhibition, 5-HT reuptake inhibition	150–400	Sedation, weight gain, dry mouth, blurry vision, constipation, urinary retention, sexual dysfunction, orthostatic hypotension, dizziness
amphetamine (psychostimulant)	Adderall, Adderall XR	NE and DA reuptake inhibition, promotes NE and DA release	5–60	Insomnia, anorexia, weight loss, irritability, tachycardia, agitation, abdominal pain, headache, dry mouth, increased psychosis, asthenia, fever, infection, growth retardation (children)
aripiprazole (antipsychotic)	Abilify	D2 partial agonist, 5-HT1A partial agonist, 5-HT2A antagonism, alpha-1 antagonism	10–30	Nausea, vomiting, headache, insomnia, somnolence, dizziness, akathisia, abnormal vision
atomoxetine (anti-ADHD)	Strattera	NE reuptake inhibition	40–100	Aggression, irritability, somnolence, vomiting, dyspepsia, nausea, fatigue, decreased appetite
benztropine (anticholinergic)	Cogentin	Anticholinergic	2–6	Tachycardia, nausea, constipation, confusion, dry mouth, urinary retention, blurry vision

GENERIC NAME (DRUG CLASS)	TRADE/BRAND NAME	MECHANISM OF ACTION	TYPICAL DOSE (MG/DAY)	MOST COMMON SIDE EFFECTS
bromocriptine (antiparkinsonian)	Parlodel	DA agonist	2.5–15	Dizziness, nausea, vomiting, dry mouth, poor appetite, abdominal pain, diarrhea, dyspepsia, constipation
buprenorphine (antiopioid)	Subutex	Partial agonist at mu-opioid receptor, antagonist at kappa-opioid receptor	2–16	Nausea, vomiting, constipation, liver dysfunction, respiratory depression
buprenorphine, naloxone (antiopioid)	Suboxone	Mixed opioid agonist-antagonist/opioid antagonist	2–16/0.5–4	Nausea, vomiting, constipation, liver dysfunction, respiratory depression, acute withdrawal syndrome
bupropion (antidepressant)	Wellbutrin, Wellbutrin SR (Zyban), Wellbutrin XL	NE reuptake inhibition, DA reuptake inhibition	75–450/ 100–400/ 150–450	Insomnia, dizziness, headache, dry mouth, nausea, decreased appetite, constipation, agitation/nervousness, seizure
buspirone (antianxiety)	Buspar	5-HT1A agonist, moderate D2 agonist	5–40	Dizziness, insomnia, nervousness, dry mouth, drowsiness, nausea, headache, fatigue
carbamazepine (mood stabilizer)	Tegretol, Tegretol XR, Carbatrol	Inhibition of sodium channels	600–1200	Nausea, vomiting, diplopia, dizziness, poor coordination, drowsiness, anemia, rash, liver dysfunction, fatigue, low WBCs
chloral hydrate (sedative–hypnotic)	Noctec	CNS depressant	500–1000	Drowsiness, dizziness, rash, confusion, restlessness, amnesia, irritability
chlordiazepoxide (antianxiety)	Librium	Increases GABA	15–40	Poor coordination, dizziness, sedation, weakness, memory dysfunction, depression, lethargy
chlordiazepoxide/ amitriptyline (antianxiety)	Limbitrol	Increases GABA, 5-HT reuptake inhibition, NE reuptake inhibition	30–60/75–150	Poor coordination, dizziness, sedation, weakness, memory dysfunction, depression, lethargy, weight gain, dry mouth, blurry vision, constipation, urinary retention, sexual dysfunction, orthostatic hypotension

GENERIC NAME (DRUG CLASS)	TRADE/BRAND NAME	MECHANISM OF ACTION	TYPICAL DOSE (MG/DAY)	MOST COMMON SIDE EFFECTS
chlorpromazine (antipsychotic)	Thorazine	D2 antagonism	200–600	Sedation, weight gain, dry mouth, dizziness, poor coordination, EPS, photosensitivity, lethargy, blurry vision, constipation, seizures, tachycardia, weakness, NMS, gynecomastia
citalopram (antidepressant)	Celexa	5-HT reuptake inhibition	10–60	Nausea, diarrhea, dry mouth, anorexia, weight gain, sexual dysfunction, tremor, restlessness, anxiety/nervousness, insomnia, dizziness, headache
clomipramine (antidepressant)	Anafranil	5-HT reuptake inhibition, NE reuptake inhibition	100–250	Sedation, weight gain, dry mouth, blurry vision, constipation, urinary retention, sexual dysfunction, orthostatic hypotension, dizziness
clonazepam (antianxiety, mood stabilizer)	Klonopin, Klonopin Wafers	Increases GABA	0.5–4	Poor coordination, dizziness, sedation, weakness, memory dysfunction, depression, lethargy
clonidine (anti-ADHD)	Catapres, Catapres Patch	Central alpha agonist	0.1–0.3	Drowsiness, dizziness, constipation, sedation, weakness, fatigue, agitation, nausea, vomiting, sexual dysfunction, myalgias, arthralgias, hypotension
clorazepate (antianxiety)	Tranxene	Increases GABA	15–60	Poor coordination, dizziness, sedation, weakness, memory dysfunction, depression, lethargy
clozapine (antipsychotic)	Clozaril, Fazaclo	D4 antagonism, alpha 2 antagonism, H1 antagonism, 5-HT antagonism	400–600	Agranulocytosis, eosinophilia, seizures, myocarditis, dizziness, tachycardia, tremor, hyperglycemia, fever, weight gain, sedation, salivation, sweating, constipation, headache, orthostatic hypotension

GENERIC NAME (DRUG CLASS)	TRADE/BRAND NAME	MECHANISM OF ACTION	TYPICAL DOSE (MG/DAY)	MOST COMMON SIDE EFFECTS
desipramine (antidepressant)	Norpramin	NE reuptake inhibition	150–300	Sedation, weight gain, dry mouth, blurry vision, constipation, urinary retention, sexual dysfunction, orthostatic hypotension, dizziness
dexmethylphenidate (psychostimulant)	Focalin	NE reuptake inhibition, DA reuptake inhibition, promotes NE and DA release	5–40	Insomnia, anorexia, weight loss, irritability, tachycardia, agitation, abdominal pain, headache, dry mouth, increased psychosis, asthenia, fever, infection, growth retardation (children)
dextroamphetamine (psychostimulant)	Dexedrine, Dexedrine Spansules, Dextrostat	NE reuptake inhibition, DA reuptake inhibition, promotes NE and DA release	5–60	Insomnia, anorexia, weight loss, irritability, tachycardia, agitation, abdominal pain, headache, dry mouth, increased psychosis, asthenia, fever, infection, growth retardation (children)
diazepam (antianxiety)	Valium	Increases GABA	5–40	Poor coordination, dizziness, sedation, weakness, memory dysfunction, depression, lethargy
diphenhydramine (antiparkinsonian)	Benadryl	Antihistamine	25–50	Sedation, dry mouth, dizziness, nausea, nervousness, headache
disulfiram (antialcohol)	Antabuse	Acetaldehyde dehydrogenase antagonist	250–500	Drowsiness, fatigue, headache, sexual dysfunction, rash, psychotic-like reactions, liver dysfunction
donepezil (antidementia)	Aricept	Cholinesterase inhibitor	5–10	Nausea, vomiting, insomnia, diarrhea, muscle cramps, fatigue, anorexia,
doxepin (antidepressant)	Sinequan, Adapin	NE reuptake inhibition, 5-HT reuptake inhibition	150–300	Sedation, weight gain, dry mouth, blurry vision, constipation, urinary retention, sexual dysfunction, dizziness, orthostatic hypotension

GENERIC NAME (DRUG CLASS)	TRADE/BRAND NAME	MECHANISM OF ACTION	TYPICAL DOSE (MG/DAY)	MOST COMMON SIDE EFFECTS
droperidol (antipsychotic)	Inapsine	D2 antagonism	2.5–15	Sedation, weight gain, dry mouth, dizziness, poor coordination, EPS, NMS, lethargy, blurry vision, seizures, constipation, tachycardia, weakness, gynecomastia
duloxetine (antidepressant)	Cymbalta	NE reuptake inhibition, 5-HT reuptake inhibition	20–60	Nausea, hypertension, anorexia, dizziness, somnolence, insomnia, dry mouth, nervousness, sexual dysfunction, sweating
escitalopram (antidepressant)	Lexapro	5-HT reuptake inhibition	5–20	Nausea, diarrhea, dry mouth, anorexia, weight gain, sexual dysfunction, tremor, restlessness, anxiety/nervousness, insomnia, dizziness, headache
estazolam (sedative-hypnotic)	Prosom	Increases GABA	2–4	Sedation, dizziness, falling, lethargy, disorientation, amnesia
eszopiclone (sedative-hypnotic)	Lunesta	Selective modulation of GABA receptor complex	2–3	Daytime drowsiness, dizziness, falls, amnesia, unpleasant taste
fluoxetine (antidepressant)	Prozac, Sarafem, Prozac Weekly	5-HT reuptake inhibition	20–80/90 (weekly)	Nausea, diarrhea, dry mouth, anorexia, weight gain, sexual dysfunction, tremor, restlessness, anxiety/nervousness, insomnia, dizziness, headache
fluoxetine, olanzepine (antidepressant/ antipsychotic)	Symbyax	Inhibition of 5-HT reuptake/DA and 5-HT2 antagonism	6–12/25–50	Asthenia, edema, increased appetite, weight gain, dry mouth, somnolence, pharyngitis, abnormal thinking, tremor
fluphenazine (antipsychotic)	Prolixin, Prolixin Decanoate	D2 antagonism	2–20/25–50 every 2 weeks	Sedation, weight gain, dry mouth, dizziness, poor coordination, EPS, NMS, lethargy, blurry vision, seizures, constipation, tachycardia, weakness, gynecomastia

GENERIC NAME (DRUG CLASS)	TRADE/BRAND NAME	MECHANISM OF ACTION	TYPICAL DOSE (MG/DAY)	MOST COMMON SIDE EFFECTS
flurazepam (sedative-hypnotic)	Dalmane	Increases GABA	15–30	Sedation, dizziness, falling, lethargy, disorientation, amnesia
fluvoxamine (antidepressant)	Luvox	5-HT reuptake inhibition	50–300	Nausea, diarrhea, dry mouth, anorexia, weight gain, sexual dysfunction, tremor, restlessness, anxiety/nervousness, insomnia, dizziness, headache
gabapentin (mood stabilizer)	Neurontin	Enhances GABA	300–3600	Dizziness, somnolence, edema, weight gain, diplopia, headache, agitation, nausea, tremors
galantamine (antidementia)	Reminyl	Cholinesterase inhibitor	16–24	Nausea, vomiting, asthenia, sweating, dizziness, headache, diarrhea, anorexia, insomnia
guanfacine (anti-ADHD)	Tenex	Central alpha agonist	0.5–3	Drowsiness, dizziness, constipation, sedation, weakness, fatigue, agitation, nausea, vomiting, sexual dysfunction, myalgias, arthralgias, hypotension
halazepam (antianxiety)	Paxipam	Increases GABA	60–160	Poor coordination, dizziness, sedation, weakness, memory dysfunction, depression, lethargy
haloperidol (antipsychotic)	Haldol, Haldol Decanoate	D2 antagonism	2–20/100–300 every month	Sedation, weight gain, dry mouth, dizziness, poor coordination, EPS, NMS, lethargy, blurry vision, seizures, constipation, tachycardia, weakness, gynecomastia
hydroxyzine (antianxiety)	Vistaril, Atarax	Antihistamine	50–150	Confusion, irritability, dry mouth, constipation, dizziness, blurry vision, sedation
imipramine (antidepressant)	Tofranil	5-HT reuptake inhibition, NE reuptake inhibition	150–300	Sedation, weight gain, dry mouth, blurry vision, constipation, urinary retention, sexual dysfunction, orthostatic hypotension, dizziness

139

GENERIC NAME (DRUG CLASS)	TRADE/BRAND NAME	MECHANISM OF ACTION	TYPICAL DOSE (MG/DAY)	MOST COMMON SIDE EFFECTS
isocarboxazid (antidepressant)	Marplan	5-HT reuptake inhibition, NE reuptake inhibition, DA reuptake inhibition	10–40	Nausea, insomnia, drowsiness, dry mouth, increased appetite, dizziness, headache, irritability, nervousness, weakness, sexual dysfunction, muscle twitching/cramps, constipation, weight gain, hypertensive crisis
L-alpha-acetyl-methadol (methadone maintenance)	LAAM	Synthetic opioid agonist	20–80 three times weekly	Feelings of unreality, hallucinations, hives, itching, rash, sweating, restlessness, nausea, vomiting, dizziness, sedation, muscle twitching, depression
lamotrigine (mood stabilizer)	Lamictal	Inhibition of sodium channels, presynaptic modulation of glutamate release	200–400	Nausea, vomiting, dizziness, diplopia, poor coordination, somnolence, headache, toxic rash
lithium carbonate or lithium citrate (mood stabilizer)	Lithobid, Eskalith CR	Enhances 5-HT, increases or decreases NE, blocks DA supersensitivity, alters second messengers	600–1200	Anorexia, dry mouth, nausea, vomiting, diarrhea, drowsiness, muscle weakness, decreased coordination, fatigue, lethargy, tremor, arrhythmias, polyuria, polydipsia, renal dysfunction, thyroid dysfunction, alopecia, rash, edema, increased appetite, weight gain
lorazepam (antianxiety)	Ativan	Increases GABA	1–6	Poor coordination, dizziness, sedation, weakness, memory dysfunction, depression, lethargy
loxapine (antipsychotic)	Loxitane	D2 antagonism	20–100	Sedation, weight gain, dry mouth, dizziness, poor coordination, EPS, photosensitivity, lethargy, blurry vision, constipation, seizures, tachycardia, weakness, NMS, gynecomastia
maprotiline (antidepressant)	Ludiomil	5-HT reuptake inhibition	150–225	Sedation, weight gain, dry mouth, blurry vision, constipation, urinary retention, sexual dysfunction, orthostatic hypotension, dizziness

GENERIC NAME (DRUG CLASS)	TRADE/BRAND NAME	MECHANISM OF ACTION	TYPICAL DOSE (MG/DAY)	MOST COMMON SIDE EFFECTS
mazindol (anticocaine)	Sanorex, Mazanor	NE reuptake inhibition, DA reuptake inhibition, promotes NE and DA release	1–3	Constipation, dizziness, dry mouth, headache, irritability, nausea, vomiting, restlessness, abdominal cramps, insomnia
memantine (antidementia)	Namenda	NMDA antagonists	10–20	Fatigue, pain, dizziness, hypertension, nausea, insomnia, flulike symptoms, edema, anxiety, anorexia, arthralgias, diarrhea, poor coordination, agitation, urinary incontinence, urinary tract infection
mesoridazine (antipsychotic)	Serentil	D2 antagonism	50–400	Sedation, weight gain, dry mouth, dizziness, poor coordination, EPS, photosensitivity, lethargy, blurry vision, constipation, seizures, tachycardia, weakness, NMS, gynecomastia
methamphetamine (psychostimulant)	Desoxyn	NE reuptake inhibition, DA reuptake inhibition, promotes NE and DA release	5–30	Insomnia, anorexia, weight loss, irritability, tachycardia, agitation, abdominal pain, headache, dry mouth, hypertension, increased psychosis, twitching
methadone (methadone maintenance)	Dolophine	Synthetic opioid agonist	20–100	Feelings of unreality, hallucinations, hives, itching, rash, sweating, restlessness, nausea, vomiting, dizziness, sedation, muscle twitching, depression
methylphenidate (psychostimulant)	Ritalin, Ritalin SR, Ritalin LA, Metadate CD, Metadate ER, Methylin Concerta	NE reuptake inhibition, DA reuptake inhibition, promotes NE and DA release	10–50	Insomnia, anorexia, weight loss, irritability, tachycardia, agitation, abdominal pain, headache, dry mouth, increased psychosis, asthenia, fever, infection, growth retardation (children)

GENERIC NAME (DRUG CLASS)	TRADE/BRAND NAME	MECHANISM OF ACTION	TYPICAL DOSE (MG/DAY)	MOST COMMON SIDE EFFECTS
mirtazepine (antidepressant)	Remeron, Remeron Soltabs	Central presynaptic alpha-2 autoreceptor antagonist, H1 antagonist, moderate alpha-1 antagonist, moderate muscarinic antagonist	15–45	Sedation, weight gain, increased appetite, dry mouth, constipation, dizziness, asthenia
modafinil (antinarcolepsy)	Provigil	DA reuptake inhibition	100–200	Headache, nausea, nervousness, rhinitis, diarrhea, back pain, insomnia, dizziness, dyspepsia
molindone (antipsychotic)	Moban	D2 antagonism	20–100	Sedation, weight gain, dry mouth, dizziness, poor coordination, EPS, photosensitivity, lethargy, blurry vision, constipation, seizures, tachycardia, weakness, NMS, gynecomastia
nalmefene (antialcohol)	Revex	Opioid antagonist	20–80	Liver dysfunction, constipation, irritability, increased thirst, dizziness, rash, chills, anorexia
naloxone (antiopioid)	Narcan	Opioid antagonist	0.4–2	Acute withdrawal syndrome, agitation, hallucinations, flushing, dyspnea, hypotension, hypertension, arrhythmias
naltrexone (antialcohol)	Revia	Opioid antagonist	50	Liver dysfunction, constipation, irritability, increased thirst, dizziness, rash, chills, anorexia, nausea, fatigue, anxiety, insomnia
nefazodone (antidepressant)	Serzone	5-HT2A antagonist	100–500	Dizziness, blurry vision, headache, dry mouth, nausea, constipation, agitation, increased appetite, drowsiness, weakness, liver toxicity
nortriptyline (antidepressant)	Pamelor, Aventyl	NE reuptake inhibition, 5-HT reuptake inhibition	75–125	Sedation, weight gain, dry mouth, blurry vision, constipation, urinary retention, sexual dysfunction, orthostatic hypotension, dizziness

GENERIC NAME (DRUG CLASS)	TRADE/BRAND NAME	MECHANISM OF ACTION	TYPICAL DOSE (MG/DAY)	MOST COMMON SIDE EFFECTS
olanzepine (antipsychotic)	Zyprexa, Zyprexa Zydis	5-HT2A and 5-HT2C antagonism, D1–D4 antagonism, M1–M5 antagonism, H1 antagonism, alpha-1 antagonism	10–20	Weight gain, increased appetite, constipation, agitation, dizziness, dry mouth, sedation, abnormal gait, back pain, speech disorder, amnesia, tremor, weakness
ondansetron (anticraving)	Zofran	5-HT3 antagonist	8–24	Diarrhea, headache, constipation, rash, dizziness, dry mouth, drowsiness
orlistat (antiobesity)	Xenical	Reversible lipase inhibitor in GI tract	360	Oily spotting or stool, flatus, fecal urgency, increased defecation, fecal incontinence
oxazepam (antianxiety)	Serax	Increases GABA	30–120	Poor coordination, dizziness, sedation, weakness, memory dysfunction, depression, lethargy
oxcarbazepine (mood stabilizer)	Trileptal	Inhibition of sodium channels, modulation of calcium channels	600–1500	Dizziness, somnolence, diplopia, nausea, vomiting, headache, ataxia, abnormal vision, abdominal pain, tremor
paroxetine (antidepressant)	Paxil, Paxil CR	5-HT reuptake inhibition	20–50/25–75	Nausea, diarrhea, dry mouth, anorexia, weight gain, sexual dysfunction, tremor, restlessness, anxiety/nervousness, insomnia, dizziness, headache
pemoline (psychostimulant)	Cylert	DA mechanisms (??)	37.5–112.5	Liver dysfunction, agitation, seizures, insomnia, anorexia, weight loss
perphenazine (antipsychotic)	Trilafon	D2 antagonism	8–64	Sedation, weight gain, dry mouth, dizziness, poor coordination, EPS, photosensitivity, lethargy, blurry vision, constipation, seizures, tachycardia, weakness, NMS, gynecomastia

GENERIC NAME (DRUG CLASS)	TRADE/BRAND NAME	MECHANISM OF ACTION	TYPICAL DOSE (MG/DAY)	MOST COMMON SIDE EFFECTS
perphenazine/ amitriptyline (antianxiety)	Triavil	D2 antagonism, 5-HT reuptake inhibition, NE reuptake inhibition	5-6-16/ 75-200	Sedation, weight gain, dry mouth, dizziness, poor coordination, EPS, photosensitivity, lethargy, blurry vision, constipation, seizures, tachycardia, weakness, NMS, gynecomastia, urinary retention, sexual dysfunction,
phenelzine (antidepressant)	Nardil	5-HT reuptake inhibition, NE reuptake inhibition, DA reuptake inhibition	30-90	Nausea, insomnia, drowsiness, dry mouth, increased appetite, dizziness, headache, irritability, nervousness, weakness, sexual dysfunction, muscle twitching/cramps, constipation, weight gain, hypertensive crisis
phentermine (antiobesity)	Adipex-P, Ionamin	NE reuptake inhibition, DA reuptake inhibition, promotes NE and DA release	37.5-75	Insomnia, anorexia, weight loss, irritability, tachycardia, agitation, abdominal pain, headache, dry mouth, increased psychosis, asthenia, fever, infection, growth retardation (children)
pimozide (antipsychotic)	Orap	D2 antagonism	1-10	Sedation, weight gain, dry mouth, dizziness, poor coordination, EPS, lethargy, NMS, blurry vision, seizures, constipation, tachycardia, weakness, gynecomastia
pramipexole (antiparkinsonian)	Mirapex	DA agonist	1.5-4.5	Nausea, dizziness, somnolence, insomnia, constipation, confusion, asthenia, hallucinations, edema, sedation, headache
prazepam (antianxiety)	Centrax	Increases GABA	20-60	Poor coordination, dizziness, sedation, weakness, memory dysfunction, depression, lethargy

GENERIC NAME (DRUG CLASS)	TRADE/BRAND NAME	MECHANISM OF ACTION	TYPICAL DOSE (MG/DAY)	MOST COMMON SIDE EFFECTS
propranolol (antianxiety) (antiparkinsonian)	Inderal, Inderal LA	Nonselective beta-blocker	20–80	Bradycardia, rash, hypotension, dizziness, depression, weakness, bronchospasm, fatigue, sexual dysfunction, insomnia, alopecia
protriptyline (antidepressant)	Vivactil	NE reuptake inhibition, 5-HT reuptake inhibition	15–60	Sedation, weight gain, dry mouth, blurry vision, constipation, urinary retention, sexual dysfunction, orthostatic hypotension, dizziness
quazepam (sedative-hypnotic)	Doral	Increases GABA	7.5–15	Sedation, dizziness, falling, lethargy, disorientation, amnesia
quetiapine (antipsychotic)	Seroquel	5-HT1A and 5-HT2 antagonism, D1 and D2 antagonism, H1 antagonism, alpha-1 and alpha-2 antagonism	300–600	Sedation, dizziness, dry mouth, asthenia, constipation, headache, liver dysfunction, weight gain, dyspepsia, orthostatic hypotension
risperidone (antipsychotic)	Risperdal, Risperdal M-tab, Risperdal Consta	D2 antagonism, 5-HT2 antagonism, alpha-1 and alpha-2 antagonism, H1 antagonism	3–6/25–50 (2 weeks)	Somnolence, EPS, weight gain, anxiety, restlessness, insomnia, dizziness, constipation, nausea, rhinitis, rash, tachycardia, sexual dysfunction
rivastigmine (antidementia)	Exelon	Cholinesterase inhibitor	6–12	Nausea, vomiting, asthenia, sweating, dizziness, headache, diarrhea, anorexia, insomnia
selegiline (antidepressant)	Eldepryl	5-HT reuptake inhibition, NE reuptake inhibition, DA reuptake inhibition	10–20	Nausea, hallucinations, insomnia, dizziness, confusion, poor balance, agitation, syncope, hypertensive crisis (higher doses)
sertraline (antidepressant)	Zoloft	5-HT reuptake inhibition	50–200	Nausea, diarrhea, dry mouth, anorexia, weight gain, sexual dysfunction, tremor, restlessness, anxiety/nervousness, insomnia, dizziness, headache

GENERIC NAME (DRUG CLASS)	TRADE/BRAND NAME	MECHANISM OF ACTION	TYPICAL DOSE (MG/DAY)	MOST COMMON SIDE EFFECTS
sibutramine (antiobesity)	Meridia	NE reuptake inhibition, 5-HT reuptake inhibition, DA reuptake inhibition	10–15	Headache, back pain, constipation, anorexia, dry mouth, dizziness, insomnia, nervousness, rhinitis, pharyngitis
tacrine (antidementia)	Cognex	Cholinesterase inhibitor	40–160	Abdominal pain, anxiety, agitation, poor coordination, constipation, depression, diarrhea, dizziness, fatigue, flushing, headache, insomnia, dyspepsia, liver dysfunction, muscle pain, anorexia, nausea, rash, sedation
temazepam (sedative-hypnotic)	Restoril	Increases GABA	15–30	Sedation, dizziness, falling, lethargy, disorientation, amnesia
thioridazine (antipsychotic)	Mellaril	D2 antagonism	200–600	Sedation, weight gain, dry mouth, dizziness, poor coordination, EPS, photosensitivity, lethargy, blurry vision, constipation, seizures, tachycardia, weakness, NMS, gynecomastia
thiothixene (antipsychotic)	Navane	D2 antagonism	5–30	Sedation, weight gain, dry mouth, dizziness, poor coordination, EPS, NMS, lethargy, blurry vision, seizures, constipation, tachycardia, weakness, gynecomastia
tiagabine (mood stabilizer)	Gabitril	Increases GABA	8–16	Dizziness, asthenia, somnolence, nausea, nervousness, abdominal pain, decreased concentration, tremor, poor coordination
topiramate (mood stabilizer)	Topamax	Increases GABA, blocks glutamate receptors	100–500	Somnolence, fatigue, dizziness, decreased weight, poor coordination, speech problems, memory dysfunction, abnormal vision, paresthesias, nervousness, confusion, cognitive dulling, headache

GENERIC NAME (DRUG CLASS)	TRADE/BRAND NAME	MECHANISM OF ACTION	TYPICAL DOSE (MG/DAY)	MOST COMMON SIDE EFFECTS
tranylcypromine (antidepressant)	Parnate	5-HT reuptake inhibition, NE reuptake inhibition, DA reuptake inhibition	20–60	Nausea, insomnia, drowsiness, dry mouth, increased appetite, dizziness, headache, irritability, nervousness, weakness, sexual dysfunction, muscle twitching/cramps, constipation, weight gain, hypertensive crisis
triazolam (sedative-hypnotic)	Halcion	Increases GABA	0.25–0.5	Sedation, dizziness, falling, lethargy, disorientation, amnesia
trifluoperazine (antipsychotic)	Stelazine	D2 antagonism	5–30	Sedation, weight gain, dry mouth, dizziness, poor coordination, EPS, NMS, lethargy, blurry vision, seizures, constipation, tachycardia, weakness, gynecomastia
trihexyphenidyl (anticholinergic)	Artane	Anticholinergic	5–15	Tachycardia, nausea, constipation, confusion, dry mouth, urinary retention, blurry vision
trimipramine (antidepressant)	Surmontil	NE reuptake inhibition, 5-HT reuptake inhibition	150–300	Sedation, weight gain, dry mouth, blurry vision, constipation, urinary retention, sexual dysfunction, orthostatic hypotension, dizziness
valproate or valproic acid (mood stabilizer)	Depakote, Depakote ER	Inhibition of sodium and/or calcium channels, increases GABA, reduces glutamate	500–2000	Nausea, vomiting, diarrhea, weight gain, abdominal pain, flatulence, edema, rash, drowsiness, tiredness, liver dysfunction, alopecia
venlafaxine (antidepressant)	Effexor, Effexor XR	NE reuptake inhibition, 5-HT reuptake inhibition	50–300/ 75–300	Nausea, hypertension, anorexia, dizziness, somnolence, insomnia, dry mouth, nervousness, sexual dysfunction, sweating

GENERIC NAME (DRUG CLASS)	TRADE/BRAND NAME	MECHANISM OF ACTION	TYPICAL DOSE (MG/DAY)	MOST COMMON SIDE EFFECTS
verapamil (mood stabilizer)	Verelan PM, Covera-HS, Isoptin SR	Calcium channel antagonist	200–400	Constipation, nausea, headache, infection, dizziness, edema, liver dysfunction, arrhythmias, rash, hypotension, fatigue
zaleplon (sedative-hypnotic)	Sonata	Selective modulation of GABA receptor complex	5–10	Daytime drowsiness, dizziness, falls, amnesia
ziprasidone (antipsychotic)	Geodon	D2 antagonism, 5-HT2 antagonism, H1 antagonism, alpha-1 antagonism	80–160	Nausea, agitation, rash, EKG abnormality, asthenia, orthostatic hypotension, anorexia, arthralgias, anxiety, tremor, rhinitis, abnormal vision
zolpidem (sedative-hypnotic)	Ambien	Selective modulation of GABA receptor complex	5–10	Daytime drowsiness, dizziness, falls, amnesia
zonisamide (mood stabilizer)	Zonegran	Inhibition of sodium and/or calcium channels, facilitates DA and 5-HT neurotransmission	200–400	Somnolence, anorexia, weight loss, dizziness, headache, nausea, agitation, mental slowing

BIBLIOGRAPHY

American Obesity Association. AOA fact sheets. www.obesity.org

American Psychiatric Association. (1994). *The diagnostic and statistical manual of mental disorders* (4th ed.-TR). Washington DC: Author.

American Psychiatric Association Clinical Resources. Practice guideline for the treatment of patients with eating disorders. www.psych.org

Antai-Otong, D. (2001). *Psychiatric emergencies: How to accurately assess and manage the patient in crisis.* Eau Claire, WI: PESI Healthcare, LLC.

Ables, A. & Baughman, O. (2003). Antidepressants: Update on new agents and indications. *American Family Physician, 67,* 547–554.

Adler, L. & Chua, H. (2002). Management of ADHD in adults. *Journal of Clinical Psychiatry, 63,* suppl 12, 29–35.

Agras, W. (2001). The consequences and costs of the eating disorders. *Psychiatric Clinics of North America, 24,* 371–379.

Aisen, P. S. (2002). The potential of anti-inflammatory drugs for the treatment of Alzheimer's disease. *Lancet Neurology, 1*(5), 279–284. Review.

Albucher, R. & Liberzon, I. (2002). Psychopharmacological treatment in PTSD: A critical review. *Journal of Psychiatric Research, 36,* 355–367.

Allen, M., Currier, G., Hughes, D., Reyes-Harde, M., & Docherty, J. (2001). Treatment of behavioral emergencies. *Postgraduate Medicine,* May 2001, Special Report.

Aviram, R., Rhum, M., & Levin, F. (2001). Psychotherapy of adults with comorbid attention deficit/hyperactivity disorder and psychoactive substance abuse disorder. *Journal Psychotherapy Practice Research, 10,* 179–186.

Baethge, C. (2002). Long-term treatment of schizoaffective disorder: Review and recommendations. *Pharmacopsychiatry, 36,* 45–56.

Barkin, R., Schwer, W., & Barkin, S. (1999). Recognition and management of depression in primary care: A focus on the elderly. A pharmacologic overview of the selection process among the traditional and new antidepressants. *American Journal of Therapeutics, 7,* 205–226.

Barkley, R. (2002). Psychosocial treatments for attention-deficit/hyperactivity disorder in children. *Journal of Clinical Psychiatry, 63,* (suppl 12), 36–43.

Bays, H. (2004). Current and investigational antiobesity agents and obesity therapeutic treatment targets. *Obesity Research, 12(8),* 1197–2211.

Bemporad, J. (2001). Aspects of psychotherapy with adults with attention deficit disorder. *Annals of New York Academy of Science, 931,* 302–309.

Bergh, C., Ejderhamn, J., & Sodersten, P. (2003). What is the evidence basis for existing treatments of eating disorders? *Current Opinion in Pediatrics, 15,* 344–345.

Bezchlibnyk-Butler, K. & Jeffries, J. (2002). *Clinical handbook of psychotropic drugs.* Seattle, WA: Hogrefe & Huber.

Bischofs, S., Zelenka, M., & Sommer C. (2004). Evaluation of topiramate as an antihyperalgesic and neuroprotective agent in the peripheral nervous system. *Journal of the Peripheral Nervous System, 9*(2), 70–78.

Blazer, D., Steffens, D., & Busse, E. (2004). *Textbook of geriatric psychiatry* (3rd ed.). Washington, DC: American Psychiatric Publishing, Inc.

Bloomfield, H., Nordfors, M., & McWilliams, P. (1996). *Hypericum and depression.* Los Angeles: Prelude Press.

Boeve, B., Silber, M., & Ferman, T. (2002). Current management of sleep disturbance in dementia. *Current Neurology and Neuroscience Reports, 2*, 169–177.

Bourin, M., & Lambert, O. (2002). Pharmacotherapy of anxious disorders. *Human Psychopharmacology, 17*, 383–400.

Bowden, C. (2001). Novel treatments for bipolar disorder. *Expert Opinion on Investigational Drugs, 10*(4), 661–671.

Brookmeyer, R., Gray, S., & Kawas, C. Projections of Alzheimer's disease in the United States and the public health: Impact of delaying disease onset. (1998). *American Journal of Public Health. 88*(9), 1337–1342.

Brooks, S., & Kushida, C. (2002). Recent advances in the understanding and treatment of narcolepsy. *Primary Psychiatry, 9, 8*, 30–34.

Buelow, G., Hebert, S., & Buelow, S. (2000). *Psychotherapist's resource on psychiatric medications* (2nd ed.). Belmont, CA: Brooks-Cole.

Bulik, C., Devlin B., & Bacanu, S. (2003). Significant linkage on chromosome 10p in families with bulimia nervosa. *American Journal of Human Genetics, 72*, 200–207.

Campbell, M., & Mathys, M. (2001). Pharmacologic options for the treatment of obesity. *American Journal of Health-System Pharmacy, 58(14)*, 1301–1308.

Carlson, N. (2004). *Physiology of behavior (8th ed.).* Boston: Allyn and Bacon.

Carvajal, G., Garcia, D., Sanchez, S., Velasco, M., Rueda, D., & Lucena, M. (2002). Hepatotoxicity associated with the new antidepressants. *Journal of Clinical Psychiatry. 63*(suppl 2), 135–137.

Cohen, L. (1997). Rational drug use in the treatment of depression. *Pharmacotherapy, 17*, 45–61.

Craddock, N., & Jones, I. (1999). Genetics of bipolar disorder. *Journal of Medical Genetics, 36*, 585–594.

Daniel, D., Zimbroff, D., Potkin, S., Reeves, K., Harrigan, E., & Lakshiminarayan, M. (1999). Ziprasidone 80 mg/d and 160 mg/d in the acute exacerbation of schizophrenia and schizoaffective disorder: A 6-week placebo-controlled trial. Ziprasidone study group. *Neuropsychophramacology, 20*, 491–505.

Dannon, P. (2003). Topiramate for the treatment of kleptomania: A case series and review of the literature. *Clinical Neuropharmacology, 26(1)*, 1–4.

Davidson, J. (2003). Pharmacotherapy of social phobia. *Acta Psychiatrica Scandinavic, 108*, 65–71.

Davies, P., & Maloney, A. J. (1976). Selective loss of central cholinergic neurons in Alzheimer's disease. *Lancet, 2*, 1403.

Devlin, M. (2002). Psychotherapy and medication for binge eating disorder. Abstract Plenary Session, *International Conference on Eating Disorders*, April, 25–28.

Doghramji, K. (2003). When patients can't sleep. *Current Psychiatry, 2*, 40–50.

Doody, R. (2003). Current treatments for alzheimer's disease: Cholinesterase inhibitors. *Journal of Clinical Psychiatry, 64*(suppl 9), 11–17.

Evans, K. (1990). *Dual diagnosis: Counseling the mentally ill substance user.* New York: Guilford Press.

Feldman, H., Gauthier, S., Hecker, J., Vellas, B., Subbiah, P., & Whalen, E. (2001). Donepezil: MSAD Study Investigators Group. A 24-week, randomized, double-blind study of donepezil in moderate to severe Alzheimer's disease. *Neurology, 57*(4), 613–620.

Gitlin, M. (1996). *The psychotherapist's guide to psychopharmacology* (2nd ed.). New York: The Free Press.

Gold, L. (2003). Psychopharmacologic treatment of depression during pregnancy. *Current Woman's Health Reports. 3*, 236–241.

Goldberg, R. (2002). Management of behavioral complications of dementia. *Medicine and Health/Rhode Island, 85* (9), 281–285.

Goodwin, F. (2002). Rationale for long-term treatment of bipolar disorder and evidence for long-term lithium treatment. *Journal of Clinical Psychiatry, 63*(suppl 10), 5–12.

Gorman, J. (2002). Treatment of generalized anxiety disorder. *Journal of Clinical Psychiatry, 63*(suppl 8), 17–23.

Grant, J., Kim, S., & Potenza, M. (2003). Advances in the pharmacological treatment of pathological gambling. *Journal of Gambling Studies, 19(1)*, 85–109.

Grant, J. & Potenza, M. (2004). Impulse control disorders: Clinical characteristics and pharmacological management. *Annals of Clinical Psychiatry, 16(1)*, 27–34.

Grossberg, G. (2003). Diagnosis and treatment of Alzheimer's disease. *Journal of Clinical Psychiatry, 64*(suppl 9), 3–6.

Grothe, D., Scheckner, B., & Albano, D. (2004). Treatment of pain syndromes with venlafaxine. *Pharmacotherapy, 24*(5), 621–629.

Grunze, H., Schlosser, S., & Walden, J. (2000). New perspectives in the acute treatment of bipolar depression. *World Journal of Biological Psychiatry, 1*, 129–136.

Halpern, A. & Mancini, M. (2003). Treatment of obesity: An update on anti-obesity medications. *Obesity Research, 4(1)*, 25–42.

Hayashida, M. & Nakane, Y. (1999). Algorithm for the treatment of acute psychotic episodes. *Psychiatry and Clinical Neurosciences, 53*(suppl), S3–S7.

Howard, K., Kopta, M., Krause, M., & Orlinsky, D. (1986). The dose response relationship in psychotherapy. *American Psychologist, 41*, 159–164.

Huxley, N., Rendall, M., & Sederer, L. (2000). Psychosocial treatments in schizophrenia. *The Journal of Nervous and Mental Disease, 188* (4), 187–201.

Insel, T. (1992). Toward a neuroanatomy of obsessive-compulsive disorder. *Archives of General Psychiatry, 49*, 739–744.

International Association for the Study of Pain. Definition of pain. www.iasp-pain.org

Janicak, P., Davis, J., Preskorn, S., & Ayd, F. (1993). *Principles and practice of psychopharmacotherapy.* Baltimore: Williams and Wilkins.

Jenike, M. (2001). An update on obsessive-compulsive disorder. *Bulletin of the Menninger Clinic. 65* (No.1), 4–25.

Jullien, R. (2001). *A Primer of drug action* (9th ed.). New York: Worth Publishers

Kane, J., Leucht, S., Carpenter, D., & Docherty, J. (2003). Introduction: Methods, commentary, and summary. *Journal of Clinical Psychiatry, 64*(suppl 12), 1–100.

Kasckow, J. (2002). Cognitive enhancers for dementia: Do they work? *Current Psychiatry, 1*(3), 22–28.

Kaye, W., Nagata, T., & Weltzin, T. (2001). Double-blind placebo-controlled administration of fluoxetine in restricting and purging-type anorexia nervosa. *Biological Psychiatry, 49*, 644–652.

Kaylor, L. (1999). Antisocial personality disorder: Diagnostic, ethical, and treatment issues. *Issues in Mental Health Nursing, 20*, 247–258.

Kelly, K. & Zisselman M. (2000). Update on electroconvulsive therapy (ECT) in older adults. *Journal of the American Geriatrics Society, 48(5)*, 560–566.

Kendell, R. E. & Adams, W. (1991). Unexplained fluctuations in the risk for schizophrenia by month and year of birth. *British Journal of Psychiatry, 158,* 758–763.

Kennedy, S., Lam, R., Cohen, N., Ravindran, A., & CANMAT Depression Work Group. (2001). Clinical guidelines for the treatment of depressive disorders IV: Medications and other biological treatments. *The Canadian Journal of Psychiatry, 46,* 38S–58S.

Klein, E., Kreinin, I., Chistyakov, A., Koren, D., Mecz, L., Marmur, S., Ben-Shachar, D., & Feinsod, M. (1999). Therapeutic efficacy of right prefrontal slow repetitive transcranial magnetic stimulation in major depression: A double-blind controlled study. *Archives of General Psychiatry, 56*(4), 315–320.

Kollins, S. (2003). Comparing the abuse potential of methylphenidate versus other stimulants: A review of available evidence and relevance to the ADHD patient. *Journal of Clinical Psychiatry, 64*(suppl 11), 14–18.

Kramer, P. (1993). *Listening to prozac.* New York: Penguin.

Kratochvil, C., Vaughan, B., Harrington, M., & Burke, W. (2003). Atomoxetine: A selective noradrenaline reuptake inhibitor for the treatment of attention-deficit/hyperactivity disorder. *Expert Opinions in Pharmacotherapy, 4*(7), 1165–1174.

Kroenke, K. (2003). Patients presenting with somatic complaints: Epidemiology, psychiatric comorbidity and management. *International Journal of Methods in Psychiatric Research, 12*(1), 34–43.

Kupfer, D. & Frank, E. (2003). Comorbidity in depression. *Acta Psychiatrica Scandinavica, 108*(suppl. 418), 57–60.

Lambert, M., Conus, P., Lambert, T., & McGorry, P. (2003). Pharmacotherapy of first-episode psychosis. *Expert Opinions in Pharmacotherapy, 4*(5), 717–750.

Le Bars, P. L., Katz, M. M., Berman, N., Itil, T. M., Freedman, A. M., & Schatzberg, A. F. (1997). A placebo-controlled, double-blind, randomized trial of an extract of ginko biloba for dementia. North American EGb Study Group. *Journal of the American Medical Association. 278*(16), 1327–1332.

Leon, A. C., Solomon, D. A., Mueller, T. I., Endicott, J., Rice, J. P., Maser, J. D., Coryell, W., & Keller, M. B. (2003). A 20-year longitudinal observational study of somatic antidepressant treatment effectiveness. *American Journal of Psychiatry, 160*(4), 727–733.

Lesperance, F., Frasure-Smith, N., & Talajic, M. (1996). Major depression before and after myocardial infarction. Its nature and consequences. *Psychosomatic Medicine, 58,* 99–110.

Lewis, M. (2002). *Child and adolescent psychiatry: A comprehensive textbook* (3rd ed.). Philadelphia: Lippincott Williams & Wilkins.

Lindesay, J. (1991). Phobic disorders in the elderly. *British Journal of Psychiatry. 159,* 531–541.

Lipsey, M. & Wilson, D. (1993). The efficacy of psychological, educational, and behavioral treatment. *American Psychologist, 48,* 1181–1209.

Livesley, W. (2000). A Practical approach to the treatment of patients with borderline personality disorder. *The Psychiatric Clinics of North America, 23*(1), 211–232.

Malhi, G., Mitchell, P., & Salim, S. (2003). Bipolar depression: Management options. *CNS Drugs, 17*(1), 9–25.

Marlatt, G.A., & Witkiewitz, K. (2002). Harm reduction approaches to alcohol use: Health promotion, prevention, and treatment. *Addictive Behaviors, 27,* 867–886.

McCann, B., & Roy-Byrne, P. (2000). Attention-deficit/hyperactivity disorder and learning disabilities in adults. *Seminars in Clinical Neuropsychiatry, 5*(3), 191–197

McIntyre, R., Muller, A., Mancini, D, & Silver, E. (2003). What to do if an antidepressant fails? *Canadian Family Physician, 49,* 449–457.

Mehler, P. (2003). Clinical practice. Bulimia nervosa. *The New England Journal of Medicine, 349,* 9, 875–881.

Merskey, H. (1979). Pain terms: A list with definitions and notes on usage. Recommended by the International Association for the Study of Pain (IASP) Subcommittee on Taxonomy. *Pain, 6,* 249–252.

Milkman, H. & Sunderwirth, S. (1987). *Craving for ecstasy.* Lexington, MA: Lexington Books.

Mintzer, J. (2001). Underlying mechanisms of psychosis and aggression in patients with Alzheimer's disease. *Journal of Clinical Psychiatry, 62* (suppl 21), 23–25.

Mintzer, J. (2003). The search for better noncholinergic treatment options for Alzheimer's disease. *Journal of Clinical Psychiatry, 64*(suppl 9), 18–22.

Mitchell, J., de Zwaan, M., & Roerig, J. (2003). Drug therapy for patients with eating disorders. *Current Drug Targets: CNS and Neurological Disorders, 1,* 17–29.

Mitchell, J., Peterson, C., Myers, T., & Wonderlich, S. (2001). Combining pharmacotherapy and psychotherapy in the treatment of patients with eating disorders. *Psychiatric Clinics of North America, 24,* 315–323.

Moller, H. & Nasrallah, H. (2003). Treatment of bipolar disorder. *Journal of Clinical Psychiatry, 64* (suppl 6), 9–17.

Mufson, M. (1999). What is the role of psychiatry in the management of chronic pain? *The Harvard Mental Health Letter, 16 (3),* 8.

Nace, E. (1992). Emerging concepts in dual diagnosis. *The Counselor, 10,* 10–13.

Nieoullon, A. (2002). Dopamine and the regulation of cognition and attention. *Progress in Neurobiology, 67,* 53–83.

Olvera, R. (2002). Intermittent explosive disorder: Epidemiology, diagnosis and management. *CNS Drugs, 16(8),* 517–26.

Oxenkrug, G., & Requintina, P. (2003). Melatonin and jet lag syndrome: Experimental model and clinical implications. *CNS Spectrums, 8*(2), 139–148.

Padwal, R., Li, S., & Lau, D. (2003). Long-term pharmacotherapy for obesity and overweight. *Cochrane Database of Systemic Reviews, 4,* CD004094.

Pearlstein, T. (2000). Antidepressant treatment of posttraumatic stress disorder. *Journal of Clinical Psychiatry, 61*(suppl 7), 40–43.

Pederson, K., Roerig, J., & Mitchell J. (2003). Towards the pharmacotherapy of eating disorders. *Expert Opinion on Pharmacotherapy, 10,* 1659–1678.

Pietrzak, R., Ladd, G., & Petry, N. (2003). Disordered gambling in adolescents: Epidemiology, diagnosis, and treatment. *Paediatric Drugs, 5(9),* 583–595.

Preston, J., & Johnson, J. (2004). *Psychopharmacology made ridiculously simple* (5th ed.). Miami, FL: Medmaster Inc.

Preston, J., O'Neal, J., & Talaga, M. (2002). *Handbook of clinical psychopharmacology for therapists* (3rd ed.). Oakland, CA: New Harbinger Publications Inc.

Pridmore, S., Oberoi, G., & Harris, N. (2001). Psychiatry has much to offer for chronic pain. *Australian and New Zealand Journal of Psychiatry, 35,* 145–149.

Prudic, J., Fitzsimons, L., Nobler, M. S., & Sackeim, H. A. (1999). Naloxone in the prevention of the adverse cognitive effects of ECT: A within-subject, placebo controlled study. *Neuropsychopharmacology. 21*(2), 285–293.

Pryse-Phillips, W., Sternberg, S., Rochon, P., Naglie, G., Strong, H., & Feightner, J. (2001). The use of medications for cognitive enhancement. *Canadian Journal of Neurological Sciences, 28*(suppl 1), 108–114.

Psychopharmacology update (2003, November). *Copy Editor, 13*(11), 1.

Raine, A. (2002). Biosocial studies of antisocial and violent behavior in children and adults: A review. *Journal of Abnormal Child Psychology, 30*(4), 311–326.

Rakel, R. (1999). Depression. *Mental Health, 26*(2), 211–224.

Reich, J. (2002). Drug treatment of personality disorder traits. *Psychiatric Annals, 32*(10), 590–596.

Reich, J. (2003). The effect of axis II disorders on the outcome of treatment of anxiety and unipolar depressive disorders: A review. *Journal of Personality Disorders, 17*(5), 387–405.

Reiger, D., Farmer, M., Rae, D., Locke, B., Keith, S., Judd, L., & Goodwin, F. (1990). Comorbidity of mental disorders with alcohol and other drugs of abuse. *Journal of the American Medical Association. 264,* 2511–2518.

Richert, A., & Baran, A. (2003). A Review of common sleep disorders. *CNS Spectrums, 8*(2), 102–109.

Rogers, S. L. & Friedhoff, L. T. (1996). The efficacy and safety of donepezil in patients with Alzheimer's disease: Results of a U.S. multicenter, randomized, double-blind, placebo-controlled trial. The donepezil study group. *Dementia, 7*(6), 293–303.

Sachs, G., Koslow, C., & Ghaemi, S. (2000). The treatment of bipolar depression. *Bipolar Disorders, 2,* 256–260.

Sachs, G., Printz, D., Kahn, D., Carpenter, D., & Docherty, J. (2000). Medication treatment of bipolar disorder 2000. *A Postgraduate Medicine Special Report,* 1–104.

Sachs, G. & Rush, J. (2003). Response, remission, and recovery in bipolar disorders: What are the realistic treatment goals? *Journal of Clinical Psychiatry, 64* (suppl 6), 18–22.

Sadock, B. & Sadock, V. (2000). *Kaplan & Sadock's comprehensive textbook of psychiatry* (7th ed.). Philadelphia: Lippincott Williams & Wilkins.

Sajatovic, M. (2003). Treatment of mood and anxiety disorders: Quetiapine and aripiprazole. *Current Psychiatry Reports, 5,* 320–326.

Sano, M. (2003). Noncholinergic treatment options for Alzheimer's disease. *Journal of Clinical Psychiatry, 64* (suppl 9), 23–28.

Sano, M., Ernesto, C., Thomas, R. G., Klauber, M. R., Schafer, K., Grundman, M., Woodbury, P., Growdon, J., Cotman, C. W., Pfeiffer, E., Schneider, L. S., & Thal, L. J. (1997). A controlled trial of selegiline, alpha-tocopherol, or both as treatment for Alzheimer's disease. The Alzheimer's disease cooperative study. *New England Journal of Medicine, 336*(17), 1216–1222.

Sattar, S., & Bhatia, S. (2003). Benzodiazepines for substance users? *Current Psychiatry, 2*(5), 25–32.

Scharf, M. (2001). Individualizing therapy for early, middle-of-the-night and late-night insomnia. *IJCP Supplement, 116,* 20–24.

Schatzberg, A., Cole, J., & DeBattista, C. (1997) *Manual of clinical psychopharmacology* (3rd ed.). Washington DC: American Psychiatric Press.

Schatzberg, A. & Nemeroff, C. (2004). *Textbook of psychopharmacology* (3rd ed.). Washington DC: American Psychiatric Press.

Schneider, J. & Irons, R. (2001). Assessment and treatment of addictive sexual disorders: Relevance for chemical dependency relapse. *Substance Use and Misuse, 36*(13), 1795–1820.

Segal, Z., Kennedy, S., Cohen, N., Group CDW. (2000). Combining psychotherapy and pharmacotherapy. *Canadian Journal of Psychiatry, 46*(suppl 1), 59S–62S.

Sekula, L., DeSantis, J., & Gianetti, V. (2003). Considerations in the management of the patient with comorbid depression and anxiety. *Journal of the American Academy of Nurse Practitioners, 15*(1), 23–33.

Sheehan, D. (1999). Venlafaxine extended release (XR) in the treatment of generalized anxiety disorder. *Journal of Clinical Psychiatry, 60*(suppl 22), 23–28.

Sheehan, D. (2001). Attaining remission in generalized anxiety disorder: Venlafaxine extended release comparative data. *Journal of Clinical Psychiatry, 62* (suppl 19), 26–31.

Sheehan, D. (2002). The management of panic disorder. *Journal of Clinical Psychiatry, 63* (suppl 14), 17–21.

Sinacola, R. (1997). Clinical psychopharmacology: The basics for licensed professional counselors. *Michigan Journal of College Student Development, 2*(1), 15–22.

Sinacola, R. (1998). The use of therapeutic assistants in outpatient psychotherapy. *Psychotherapy in Private Practice, 17*(3), 35–44.

Singh, Y. & Singh, N. (2002). Therapeutic potential of kava in the treatment of anxiety disorders. *CNS Drugs, 16*(11), 731–743.

Sonawalla, S. B., & Fava, M. (2001). Severe depression: Is there a best approach? *CNS Drugs. 15*(10), 765–776. Review.

Sonawalla, S. B. & Fava, M. (2001). Severe depression: Is there a best approach? *CNS Drugs, 15*(10), 765–776.

Sood, E., Pallanti, S., & Hollander, E. (2003). Diagnosis and treatment of pathological gambling. *Current Psychiatry Reports, 5(1),* 9–15.

Spencer, T., Biederman, J., Wilens, T., & Faraone, S. (2002). Overview and neurobiology of attention-deficit/hyperactivity disorder. *Journal of Clinical Psychiatry, 63* (suppl 12), 3–9.

Stahl, S. (1997). *Psychopharmacology of antidepressants.* London: Martin Dunitz.

Stahl, S. (2001). *Essential psychopharmacology of depression and bipolar disorder.* New York: Cambridge University Press.

Strachey, J. (1953). On the physical mechanisms of hysterical phenomena (1893). *The standard edition of the complete psychological works of Sigmund Freud, 3,* 25–42.

Sullivan, H. (1953). *Conceptions of modern psychiatry.* New York: Norton.

Suppes, T., Dennehy, E., Swann, A., Bowden, C., Calabrese, J., Hirschfeld, R., Keck, P., Sachs, G., Crismon, M., Toprac, M., & Shon, S. (2002). Report of the Texas Consensus Conference Panel on Medication Treatment of Bipolar Disorder 2000. *Journal of Clinical Psychiatry, 63*(4), 288–299.

Sutherland, J., Sutherland, S., & Hoehns, J. (2003). Achieving the best outcome in treatment of depression. *The Journal of Family Medicine, 52*(3), 201–209.

Swift, R. (2001). The pharmacotherapy of alcohol dependence: Clinical and economic aspects. *The Economics of Neuroscience, 3*(12), 62–66.

Tandon, R. & Jibson, M. (2003). Efficacy of newer generation antipsychotics in the treatment of schizophrenia. *Psychoneuroendocrinology, 28,* 9–26.

Tariot, P. N., Farlow, M. R., Grossberg, G. T, Graham, S. M., & McDonald Memantine Study Group. (2004). Memantine treatment in patients with moderate to severe Alzheimer's disease already receiving donepezil: A randomized controlled trial. *Journal of the American Medical Association, 291*(3), 317–324.

Triggs, W., McCoy, K., Greer, R., Rossi, F., Bowers, D., Kortenkamp, S., Nadeau, S., Heilman, K., & Goodman, W. (1999). Effects of left frontal transcranial magnetic stimulation on depressed mood, cognition, and corticomotor threshold. *Biological Psychiatry, 45,* 1440–1446.

Tyler, V. (1993). *The honest herbal* (3rd ed.). New York: Pharmaceutical Products Press/Haworth Press.

U.S. Food and Drug Administration. Proposed medication guide. www.fda.gov

van der Weide, J., Steijns, L. S., & van Weelden, M. J. (2003). The effect of smoking and cytochrome P450 CYP1A2 genetic polymorphism on clozapine clearance and dose requirement. *Pharmacogenetics, 13*(3), 169–172.

Viguera, A., Cohen, L., Baldessarini, R., & Nonacs, R. (2002). Managing bipolar disorder during pregnancy: Weighing the risk and benefits. *Canadian Journal of Psychiatry, 47*(5), 426–436.

Wadden, T., Sarwer, D., & Womble, L. (2001). Psychosocial aspects of obesity and obesity surgery. *Surgical Clinics of North America, 81,* 1004–1024.

Walsh, K. & McDougle, C. (2001). Trichotillomania. Presentation, etiology, diagnosis, and therapy. *American Journal of Clinical Dermatology, 2(5),* 327–333.

Warren M. (2004). A comparative review of the risks, and benefits of hormone replacement therapy regimens. *American Journal of Obstetrics and Gynecology, 190*(4), 1141–1167.

Weiss, L. (1992). *Attention deficit disorders in adults.* Dallas, TX: Taylor Publishing.

Weiss, M., & Murray, C. (2003). Assessment and management of attention-deficit hyperactivity disorder in adults. *Canadian Medical Association Journal, 168*(6), 715–722.

Wenk, G. (2003). Neuropathologic changes in Alzheimer's disease. *Journal of Clinical Psychiatry, 64*(suppl 9), 7–10.

Williams, J. & Hughes, J. (2003). Treatments for tobacco dependence among smokers with mental illness or addiction. *Psychiatric Annals, 33*(7), 457–466.

Wilson, J. & Levin, F. (2001). Attention deficit hyperactivity disorder (ADHD) and substance use disorders. *Current Psychiatry Reports, 3,* 497–506.

Zimmerman, M. (2003). Attention-deficit hyperactivity disorders. *Nursing Clinics of North America, 38,* 55–66.

INDEX

Note: Information presented in tables and figures is denoted by *t* or *f* respectively.